Me, You, Them

Me, You, Them

EVIE SAGE

MICHAEL 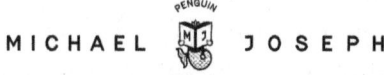 JOSEPH

PENGUIN MICHAEL JOSEPH

UK | USA | Canada | Ireland | Australia
India | New Zealand | South Africa

Penguin Michael Joseph is part of the Penguin Random House group of companies whose addresses can be found at global.penguinrandomhouse.com

Penguin Random House UK,
One Embassy Gardens, 8 Viaduct Gardens, London SW11 7BW

penguin.co.uk

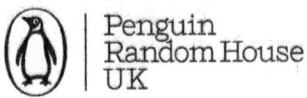

First published 2025

001

Copyright © Evie Sage, 2025

The moral right of the author has been asserted

Penguin Random House values and supports copyright.
Copyright fuels creativity, encourages diverse voices, promotes freedom of expression and supports a vibrant culture. Thank you for purchasing an authorized edition of this book and for respecting intellectual property laws by not reproducing, scanning or distributing any part of it by any means without permission. You are supporting authors and enabling Penguin Random House to continue to publish books for everyone.
No part of this book may be used or reproduced in any manner for the purpose of training artificial intelligence technologies or systems. In accordance with Article 4(3) of the DSM Directive 2019/790, Penguin Random House expressly reserves this work from the text and data mining exception

This book is a work of non-fiction based on the life, experiences and recollections of the author. The names of people, places, dates, sequences and the detail of events have been changed to protect the privacy of others

Set in 13.5/16pt Garamond MT Std
Typeset by Jouve (UK), Milton Keynes
Printed and bound in Great Britain by Clays Ltd, Elcograf S.p.A.

The authorized representative in the EEA is Penguin Random House Ireland,
Morrison Chambers, 32 Nassau Street, Dublin D02 YH68

A CIP catalogue record for this book is available from the British Library

HARDBACK ISBN: 978–0–241–73018–8

Penguin Random House is committed to a sustainable future for our business, our readers and our planet. This book is made from Forest Stewardship Council® certified paper.

To all those living outside the lines

'I feel no shame in writing these things because of the time which separates the moment when they are written – when only I can see them – from the moment when they will be read by other people, a moment which I feel will never come.'

– *Annie Ernaux,* Simple Passion

'The most terrifying thing is to accept oneself completely.'

– *C. G. Jung*

Three

2019

The first time, I'm afraid: of things falling into place, of knowing deeply that this is right. That all along I've been fighting a tide that with one wave would wipe out ordinary life.

The dullness of a shopping centre on a Tuesday afternoon seems the perfect place to start a fire.

In the car, we move too quickly along grey, wet English roads. My thoughts run fast, jarring as if needing oil. What happens if? What will we do, when? I keep these thoughts inside, smoothing the surface of my white shirt and straightened hair. I rarely wear makeup and feel unlike myself.

We've trawled for months and caught someone, claiming to be real. We've talked every angle dry; if we didn't know this maze by heart, we wouldn't risk losing our way.

We wait in Starbucks on the central concourse amongst people going about their ordinary days, with shopping bags full of unneeded things and list-filled brains.

In our minds, we hold a photo of a girl, standing on

a white balcony in a yellow dress – a sunny place, far from here.

We send a message – *We're wearing white* – and wait, wondering if she has cold feet. Rolling the thought around, I find only relief.

She arrives, bigger than her photos, and calls us names that are only ours online.

'Sorry I'm late,' she says. 'The traffic. Have you done this before?'

We shake our heads. 'We've talked about it for years.'

I look at her as she talks too fast, exposing herself to us in a way that leaves no mystery. I imagine her, driving her car in traffic, in the world out there. Every word she says brings her closer to normality, to ordinary, further from fantasy, from how I want this experience to be.

She's pleasant-looking, with long brown hair, a wide, toothy smile. I'm not drawn to her, and I wonder if I should be, if what she offers is enough.

We drink bottled water, asking small questions, avoiding the big one.

She says it, after a while.

'Shall we do this?'

We look at each other, and nod.

She's not perfect, but she'll do. I wanted this moment in a plush hotel room, high above a city, the lights glimmering below. We're breaking some glass wall I didn't know was there, and I want the sound of alarms.

We walk through near-empty corridors, pass shops whose familiarity jars. What are they doing here in this new world?

I walk behind you and this girl, struck by a thunderbolt thrill that we are doing this in broad daylight, like getting away with murder.

What will happen when we reach that room?

At the check-in desk of a Travelodge across the motorway bridge, you book a room. We listen to breakfast and check-out information as if it matters.

Soon, we're giggling in the lift, opening the door to a room with a bed. I wonder, how will it begin?

She takes my hand and leads me into the room, unbuttoning my shirt. I'm grateful that she takes control and reciprocate until we are in underwear. The mattress is there below us. I feel you, behind, taking off your clothes, then her small hot lips on mine.

'Nice tits,' she says, handling them as you join us on the bed in boxer shorts. We watch as her mouth moves between my legs and look at each other before my eyes close.

It is like coming home, like cocktails in the sun. A glimpse of some parallel female life. There is an age to it, something social, urgent, an ancientness: as if I have visited here in a dream.

Her hands travel down my body: all those whispered conversations at sleepovers, glances in the school changing room, over years begin to converge in a blistering light. I feel each nerve, fearing it will be too much. I have waited for this feeling, wondering, and now it's here I long to both contain it and exist within it, feeling its passing before it's over. Tenderly, she holds me there, inside this place that is just ours. This rising has a different flavour, a quiet calm. Your eyes on the other side of the bed bear witness.

Longing to give her what she's given me, I move my mouth, feeling her body shift like ocean waves almost as if it were my own, and a door opens to another place.

Then you move towards her. She asks if that's okay. I nod and watch you kiss her. I search myself for jealousy, but there is only strange fascination at this new thing.

She checks before taking you fully in her hand, smiling as if satisfied with what she's found. As I watch you enter her, I hear her gasp, and I feel – pride – that you are mine, the pleasure doubling with being shared.

Bent over, she is fucked. I lie beneath with fingers on her clit, feeling her panting breath, watching as she loses herself and knowing deeply what it's like.

When it's over, we lie all three on ruffled sheets. Catching our breath, waiting for the fire to pass. We kiss goodbye and promise to do this again sometime.

PART I
Beginnings

Her

2003

She's late to class again. The smell of sweet perfume; her dark hair shining under strip lights. The Tipp-Ex hearts on her school bag glow. Her skirt is the same as mine, shorter on much longer legs.

She slips into her seat, picks up the proffered earphone from her best friend, shutting out the sound of the register being called.

I sit straight at the front of the class, as though listening to the teacher, but only hearing the scratch of their pencils as they write notes.

My best friend and I are sunshine and rainbows. We not only complete our work, we decorate it too. We spend our time in stationery and craft shops, examining aisles of buttons, threads, stickers. During lunchtime breaks, we find projects in the science lab, or spend hours formatting fonts on computers in the library, keeping our voices below the required levels.

I'm magnetised by her, feeling the pull against my will.

I mask my interest with disinterest, not catching her eye when we pass alone in the halls. The first time we truly cross paths – I'm with my best friend at a disco at the local boys' school. There's a gender split on the dance floor, breached only by the bold. The best-looking boy chooses the best-looking girl. I lose myself, watching them sway under the dimmed lights, his arms around her waist. I long to be where she is, rotating in the spotlight, picked out for everyone to see. When I look up, I've lost track of my friend.

I find them outside, round the side of the building, sharing a cigarette. This is so far from the rules we live by, I feel betrayed.

'Smoking will kill you,' I say – the first words I ever say to her.

'It's only one,' my friend says, blinking like a doll shaken up and down.

'It's a slippery slope,' I say, not sure what I mean.

I can feel her grey eyes on me as I speak, appraising me with a slight smirk, as if she's putting me firmly in a box of people who are not her people. I want to stop, to grab the cigarettes out of her hand and light one. But I don't.

We travel by bus to France: endless hours of singing, crumbs, travel sickness, crick-necked sleep. I buy a croissant with a euro note at a service station, share it with my neighbour.

We arrive late at night, the weary teachers thrilled to dispose of us in bunk-bed rooms.

She and I are allocated a room together with several

mutual friends. Our best friends aren't here – neither could afford the trip.

The first night, we all stay up too late – gossiping long after lights out. I try my first cigarette out of the bedroom window, just to feel her eyes on me again. Afterwards, I brush my teeth hard. Someone brings a bottle of gin and someone else gets sick, commandeering the small bathroom. One girl strokes another girl's arm until she falls asleep.

All these things are normal here, remain a secret, and we are at breakfast as if none of it has happened. I'm startled, astounded, that the teachers don't see the marks of disobedience on our faces. It is the first time I start to see the grey areas, the hidden things.

On the slopes, I expect her to be at the front with the confident ones, the fast-movers who have been skiing since they could walk. She's on the netball team, plays hockey and runs. But on the first steep slope, the group traverse one by one, and she and I end up stuck sideways across the hill. I see us as if I am a bird swooping overhead; two black dots, surrounded by pure white.

'Just push forwards,' the impatient French teacher shouts from where the others wait.

I feel a surge of fear in my belly – I look back at her and see it mirrored in her grey-blue eyes.

At the end of the first day, he grades us, and we're the only ones who get two stars instead of three.

We take off our boots in a rubber-floored room, and I feel her beside me.

I announce I want to buy postcards from the gift shop. She offers to come. I feel the dynamics in the room shift; keeping my face smooth, I smile inside.

On the way to the cobbled square, I watch us from far away. I make her laugh and wonder who this person is, oddly proud.

We survey the rack of postcards, choosing the strangest ones of animals skiing and cartoon fish, collapsing into laughter that feels like cement, as if we're building something new and strong. I want to stop, to examine and understand, but let myself be pulled along.

'I can't believe he gave us two stars,' she says, as we wander back.

'I know,' I say.

Her eyes focus coolly, as if she's looking down crosshairs. 'We'll show him,' she says.

He is now our enemy. We pretend we can't hear him when he calls simple instructions, preferring to trace our own paths down the mountain. When we return, the tanned skin around his nose and mouth puckers, his eyes narrow. We smirk. Underneath, I feel sorry for him, but nothing is more important than maintaining her attention.

Eventually, he leaves us and focuses on the others who will listen. We spend the week larking about, pretending not to care about improvements we could easily be making. At the final ceremony when he hands out the certificates, he hands us the only two stars. We laugh behind our hands. We've gained something else this week, and for the first time, I care more about that than being the best. It's been a holiday from over-achievement, from curating perfect scores, and I don't want it to end.

On the coach home, we sit together. She plays her favourite songs, and I practise telling her what I really think, sensing that she craves challenge. We bemoan going home, complaining about our families. I feel bad, thinking about my hardworking father and caring mother, but betray them anyway.

What is it that I'm trying to gain from this, I wonder, staring out of the window as France turns to England. I look at her, side glances, and try to work it out. Her beauty makes her powerful, gives her the luxury of shrugging her shoulders, of not caring. But it's more than that: she seems to know herself. I want that. I want to be her equal.

As we re-enter England, I start to feel a heaviness descend. Once we're back at school, I'll be back with my old best friend, watching someone else take my place beside her. The thought of coloured pens and homework makes me tired and sad.

'What's wrong?' my mum asks, as I push my dinner around my plate.

I shrug, unable to find the words to explain.

'Did you not have fun?'

How can she possibly understand? 'I'm fine,' I say, more sharply than I mean.

The hurt flashes across her face, her worry like a burden, but I can't care now.

I lie awake, mourning something I never really had.

The next morning, I walk into the classroom. She's already there in her usual place. She waves me over, tells me she's got some new music to show me, offers me the ear bud. I pause, looking over at my old best friend, watching from our seats. Then I slide into the seat beside her and my new friend smiles.

Before her, there were others.

The boy who played the woodcutter in the school play. I watched him under bright sports-hall lights and longed to be Snow White.

The girl who wanted to perform in the West End, practising after school in rehearsal rooms.

The summer-camp boy. We danced to 'Eternal Flame', bodies close.

The holiday romance. An Irish boy, with braces and blonde hair. One day, he said, 'There's something I have to do,' and kissed me.

The writer girl I'd meet in coffee shops, who dressed in garish vintage clothes.

I longed to be with them, near them.

I wrote in my diary: do not accept an ordinary life.

It helps that she is pretty.

We do each other's hair, painting faces in her parents' marble bathroom. We try on versions of ourselves, wondering what tonight will bring. The unknown of dark places is intoxicating, addictive.

'You can't go out wearing that,' her dad says, as we sneak out the side door, running towards her car, cigarettes hidden in tiny handbags.

Our cars are the first place we find freedom from the rules set only out of love. We stop in a lay-by and smoke, watching fields and the edges of big houses, talking about how hard life is when we have everything and each other.

We drive along singing love songs at the tops of our voices. In her playroom, we watch *Thelma & Louise* together, bodies close under cartoon duvets pulled from childhood bedrooms, shovelling popcorn. I imagine us driving off a cliff in an open-top car, hair blowing in the wind.

'We should run away together,' she says, and I smile that she is thinking the same as me, imagining driving towards the coast, finding an anonymous town and making it ours. Creating a life where I am the person I've always hoped I could be: brave, bold, unconcerned what others think.

At the bar, we jump the snaking queue outside, calling the bouncer's name. The music thrums beneath our skin. Eyes follow us. I see us reflected in the mirrors behind the rows of glass bottles, happy to be in my body, in this place, now. She's tall, commands attention, refuses to stoop to accommodate others.

Drinks in hand, we dance too close, running our

hands on each other, our lips almost brushing. I feel a rush flow through me as I see the men watching us. Looking in her eyes and not knowing whether the feeling there is real or pretend.

I am pouting Britney dancing in the school hall, eyeballing the camera, her stomach taut and brown. I am watched and wanted.

Her boyfriend is suddenly there with his friends. He's one of the cool boys from the boys' school. The night he'd picked her, we'd been so excited. She'd spent hours choosing what to wear, nervously checking her reflection. I'd thought she didn't care about anything, but saw that she does.

That was months ago; now he's hers, she's lost interest. He's been trying to find her, and as usual, he's irritated with himself for caring more than she does. She's annoyed with him for cramping our style, for interrupting us. There's something the wrong way round about her priorities, but I'm on the right side and don't complain. Being in her light is the best feeling I have found so far, and I never want it to end.

I fantasise about kissing him sometimes. About how forbidden it would be, to feel his lips on mine. About being in one of those body-swap films, waking up in her body, being her. His friend is in love with me, but I don't want him. When he tries to kiss me, I make excuses. He's nice, good-looking, but there's something in his eagerness, his uncomplicated affection, that makes me shrug him off. I kiss boys in clubs when we go out, enjoying watching them from across the room, drawing them towards me with a simple smile. I am in control of this, or feel I am.

We escape him. Later, outside the kebab shop, we flirt with men who tease, calling us Grade A dirt as we pretend to kiss. We smile, proud of being desired, of being good and bad at once.

We walk home, buzzing with our glow. Outside the park, behind some trees, we do kiss, then break apart laughing. We do this sometimes when we're drunk, wake up in each other's arms and never speak of it again.

It feels inevitable, a logical next step, to extend the thing we're creating into a proper kiss. I want her in those moments, but this is also a way to solidify what we have, to show its depth and significance.

The next day, hungover, she rows with her parents. Slams the door, runs to her car, and I follow. I stay quiet as she reverses out of the long driveway, turns up the music and puts her foot down on the open road. I know like no one else how to handle her and I'm certain it's what makes us different. She's difficult, hard to win, and that makes her a wanted prize.

I worry deeply that I'm in love with her. Is this what love is: obsession, want? I write about it in my diary, my fear that I care more about her than she does about me. I constantly search for signs that what we have is balanced, equal. We talk about it sometimes, tell each other we love each other. But where does one love end, and another sort begin? I'm addicted to the mystery of what this thing is, wanting and not wanting for it to be the real thing. That tension hangs between us, making us who we are. If I voice the words, without subtext, I fear the horror on her face, her growing cold, and pushing me away.

At school, we both excel. On exam results day, we're photographed for national papers, clutching each other as we open envelopes with perfect results. In the photo, I wear a white fluffy jumper and jeans, my hair is straightened and I clutch at her t-shirted body with a look of genuine joy. I wonder if others can see the love in my eyes. I worry about it, then don't care. She clutches me too.

We have a double life – we sit with her parents' friends at dinner, allowed a single glass of wine. We debate the issues of the day, and hold our own. We imagine them, after we've gone to bed – such bright young things, they say to each other. After all, we are only a reflection of them.

We go out until 3am, then get up and drive to school on time. Our parents let it slide – as long as our reports glow, we must be doing fine. I feel we are untouchable, and could do anything together.

Being a teenage girl is dangerous – we push as if against a solid wall, when the world is a flimsy place that will not hold our weight.

*

The shopping centre is newly built – the place to be seen, with miles of brand-new shops, faux-marble floors and a food hall modelled on the *Titanic*'s hull. We stand at the edge imagining the wind in our hair, arms round each other, laughing as we mock real love.

We choose clothes for each other to try on, sharing a cubicle, averting eyes. I see her reflected in the mirror but pretend I don't. Her body is different to mine, and therefore fascinating. I want to see it, to compare.

She's chosen a clingy red dress for me. I pull it on, making myself look at my reflection, but only because she's there, brave because I want her to see me so. Changing rooms are places where the truth is far from what I want it to be. Bright lights engorge my thighs, make bulges where I cannot bear to look.

'You look amazing,' she says, and I try hard to believe those words, like a birthday-candle wish.

She tugs at her own skirt, and I pass her a top: a scrap of material crossed at the back with sparkly string.

'You should try this,' I say, and she shrugs, pulls off her top and bra, and puts it on.

I feel myself inhale – she's stunning, glittering, everything I would like to be.

'Wow,' I say, and she smiles, as if she knows, but needs to hear.

'We should get these,' she says, and so we do.

We've been procrastinating, eating lunch and entering every other shop, but now it's time. I hold my breath as we cross inside, where bright-coloured lingerie are candies, dripping from hangers, shimmering in the electric light. We pass it all, moving towards the darker belly of the shop, where narrow shelves hold an array of the items we have come for.

Vibrators, bold against the darkness. We glance at each other. A dark-eyed shop assistant lurks, but before she can ask excruciating questions, I find the one we've seen in magazines, the one the girls at school are talking about. We move to the counter, pay and leave the shop.

Outside, we sit on a quiet bench and pull the packaged items from the paper bag. Pink and pearled, named for a favoured pet, two Rabbits wait.

'I can't believe we've done it,' I say, and she grins wide.

We try them on our own in bedrooms hanging far above our parents' boring lives. Their takeaways and Saturday night TV seem humdrum as I pull my new toy from its box, insert the batteries, try the buttons out. Under the covers, I press the ears to my flesh, expecting slowness, mystery. Almost immediately I am transported from my mind, and eyes wide, come.

It's happened before, one evening in my locked bathroom. I held my breath, afraid of any noise, and leg up on the bath, I felt inside myself. It was a slower, softer rise, a losing of something to gain calm. My mind was clear and flat; as soon as it was over, I felt bad.

The Rabbit is quick, efficient. Part of me is not sure it's the same as when I use my fingers, that without the slow lotus-unfurling in my body I'm losing some connection with myself, but I push those thoughts down.

At school, we find a private place somewhere and talk, urgently.

'I liked it,' she says. 'Did you?'

'How could I not?'

It makes me glow, to think of us, on this secret adventure together. That we are doing something brave and bold that marks us out. If she does this and I do too, it's something sacred but also ordinary, safe, normal.

Sometimes, I think of her. I come, trembling, and immediately the shame pours in. What does it mean that she is there in dark places behind my lids?

Her and I, dancing close, our bodies touching.

Sometimes, I am inside her body, under her skin. I feel her power thrum as if it is my own, so close. I want to be seen by her, to be loved deeply by her, but also to be her.

A holiday somewhere hot, just me and her.

At the airport we check in, waving goodbye to overstuffed suitcases. The plane taxies down the runway. We marvel as the world we know becomes a toy town: green and lush, punctuated by the open sores of housing estates. I reach out and squeeze her hand. She smiles, brushing a hair out of my eye.

I hold my breath as we order gin and tonics. The air

hostess looks us over, shrugs and lays them before us. We chink, buzzing with the novelty.

We do crosswords on the plane from a book her mother gave her, laughing when we get it wrong. We scan for boys, but all the ones we find talk too loud or wear the wrong clothes; won't fit our idea of the holiday.

She isn't a fan of landings and puts her head on my shoulder, holds my arm.

It feels like we've survived something as the plane bumps down. Stepping out, the hot air rushes over our skin. The light bounces off the swathe of concrete; we pull cheap sunglasses over our faces. In the crowded bus we wrinkle our noses. At passport control, I smile, but the man doesn't look up. Soon we're out, following Spanish signs to the taxi rank, pulling out the papers my mum has printed and pointing at the name of our hotel to a man who nods then climbs into the car.

'Not exactly luxury,' she says, as we pull up outside a yellowing white facade, four storeys high, a two-star sign hanging over the mucky glass doorway.

'It'll do,' I say, and she smiles.

The room is small, the shutters pulled across patio doors that lead onto a miniature balcony. There's a kitchenette and plastic sofa, gaudy tiled floors, stiff twin beds and a bathroom with tired linoleum. It's much worse than what we're used to on family holidays, but it's ours.

She flops onto her bed, pulling her top over her head, revealing a pink bowed bra. 'It's perfect,' she says, and I agree.

We unpack our various shiny, slippery clothes into the small wardrobe and chest of drawers, heading to the shop just outside the hotel to pick up essential provisions: a six-litre carton of sangria, a bag of pasta, pasta sauce, packet ham, cheese, bread, eggs, a lonely tomato and an avocado.

Back in the room, she sets about making dinner: boiling the water for pasta, tearing up ham, pouring the sauce into a pan. She passes me the cheese and a grater.

She is used to fending for herself – the first time I went to her house for tea, her dad threw me a pepper. I found a knife, hovering it over the ripe plump thing, feeling his eyes on me. Eventually I cut it up. When I handed him the board, he smirked and redid what I had done.

At my house, I arrive home from school to delicious smells, sent off to the living room to watch TV. Sometime later a meal appears.

I pour us sangria and we chink, carrying our plates out onto the balcony.

'This is what it would be like if we had our own place,' I say.

She smiles. 'We will one day, when we move to London.'

Somewhere in the blurry future, this version of us

exists. A dusty, messy flat, strung with fairy lights and pink cushions.

I'm impatient for it, but we've been accepted to universities at opposite ends of the country. We'll be parting ways for three years. We don't talk about it apart from when we're drunk.

'Do you ever worry that no one there will like you?' I say once, slurring words.

'No,' she says. 'I worry I won't find anyone I like.'

This selectiveness seems alien to me. I can make myself like anyone, I think, filling spaces like a strange chameleon. I long to be so sure, to hold myself up truly to be seen.

'It's so warm,' I say now, holding my hand out as if the air is sunlight.

'I bet it's raining at home.'

The sun is fading in the direction of the sea, turning the sky red, tinging our faces pink. We take photos, pouting with the bottle of sangria, kissing for the camera. We can see a little version of the photos on the back of her digital camera, and we try to appraise them, but we won't really know until we return home and see them on computer screens or rush to have them developed.

We drink tart sangria, and after a few glasses it goes down well. A pigeon lands on the edge of the balcony in the fading light, cooing at us. We name her Penelope, snapping her with the camera. I can already feel we'll joke about this in years to come when we have families and kids and husbands and life isn't just us. It makes me sad to think about that, so I light another cigarette, and hers, watching her face as she concentrates on inhaling.

'We should go out,' she says. We start making preparations. She tries on top after top, dress after dress, needing the perfect outfit for the perfect night. We swap clothes. I feel different in hers, like an actress playing a role. I look at myself in the mirror, at us, side by side: complementary, two parts of something complete. She is stop-traffic good-looking: tall, statuesque, with long hair and dark features; I'm the pleasant girl next door, blonde with rosebud lips and large eyes, like a doll.

She sprays me with her perfume; I apply her lip gloss. We grab the camera, cigarettes, euros, our handbags, slip on uncomfortable shoes, and head down to reception. A family is coming back from dinner, and I feel the eyes of the father on us, pushing my breasts out, smiling, but not looking at him.

We take a taxi to the nearest bar. We meet some guys — good-looking, local — who buy us drinks and push wads of menthol tobacco into our upper gums. We look at each other, but do it anyway. When they invite us to a bigger club, we agree, and it's only when we're in a car speeding away from the hotel down a major arterial that I start to feel uneasy. We surface-laugh and sing along with the radio, but I wonder if she's panicking too. I imagine a news story about missing English girls.

When we pull up outside a huge black building lit up in neon, I smile too hard as we're waved past the queue while our companions handshake the bouncer. She loops her arms around me and squeezes; I feel our bare legs rub against each other and feel a jolt of happiness.

We all do shots at the bar. The taller, dark-haired one is wearing sunglasses inside. It doesn't hide the fact that he's looking at me. I feel his glances on my skin, as if he is applying light pressure with his hands. I stand up straighter, smile.

'He's into you,' she whispers, as we lean on the bar waiting for more cocktails to be poured.

'I know,' I say, and she laughs.

It seems irrelevant to ask if I'm into him.

We shake off the men, hit the dance floor. The music is loud and we move around each other, making a show, aware of our audience.

I feel his hands before I see him. He is dancing behind me, tracing his fingers along my waist. His blonde friend is dancing with her – he's smaller, and they look odd together. I move my hips, keeping my face still. I feel a flutter of fear as if I'm running out of time to decide if I want this. The gap between our bodies is closing. Once he kisses me, I know I will kiss him back.

I open my eyes and she's looking at me, smiling with the other guy. I lean into him, moving my hips backwards slightly. That's all it takes. He spins me round and kisses me. A good kiss, tinged with tobacco; it feels like holiday, like something I wouldn't do at home. I am not thinking about him, or me, but how this makes her feel. The thought feels wrong but right. After a while, I disentangle, laughing, running towards her, pulling us towards the bar.

We get a taxi back to the hotel, singing all the way. We have a drink and a cigarette on the terrace as the sun comes up and I think: *These are the best years of our lives.* Even as they pass by, I know this. I want to hit pause, to stay here with her forever.

'Promise me we'll always be like this,' I say.

'I promise,' she says.

Him

2007

The first time I see you, you're kissing my flatmate.

A university night out: a large blue oval bar, where bodies press and squeeze. Sweet cheap drinks and nights that never seem to end, bleeding into each other in one long colourful cascade.

You're dressed as a doctor; she's on Class As. I see you on a central seat in easy view, lips locked, and wonder what it would feel like if I was in her place. Your mouth on mine, your male taste, your tongue.

I ask someone who you are, and they tell me that you once killed a mouse with your bare hands. I am intrigued by this, feeling some magnetic draw towards something so real and raw.

You're good-looking – taller than the other boys, with broader shoulders. Film-star-like – chiselled jaw, just the right amount of stubble, piercing blue-green eyes. You have confidence, a presence, even from across the room.

She's attractive too – big breasts, long legs, coloured blonde hair, a pretty face. We've been in competition before; another boy, who'd chosen her. I spent the summer au pairing in Europe, running through woodland, trundling a wet-mouthed child around a lake, trying to forget.

The following day, I watch her check her phone, wishing she was dead. I smile as she talks of messages you've sent, smoothing my face as if icing a cake.

The next time I see you, it's at our flat. A poky, grey-stone place, a few minutes' walk from lectures. Tonight, it's rammed: my birthday party – Barbie themed – I'm dressed in a baby-pink dress, wearing a platinum wig. I've applied fake eyelashes. I've checked myself repeatedly in the mirror of the dim bathroom; smoothed skin with makeup brushes, searched the back of my head for kinked hair, terrified of missing some crucial detail which might mean the difference between being chosen and not.

You haven't come for me: she's invited you, without my say.

I'm outside as you arrive, smoking a fuck-life cigarette, pretending to be cool.

'Want one?' I say, but you shake your head. My stomach drops, feeling the darkness of a potential misstep.

I lose track of you that night; she mentions you over the weeks that follow. At first, she gloats, but soon things change. You make the mistake of being too eager – she wants the chase, and soon she is looking over your shoulder at someone else.

*

The first time we officially meet, we're at a toga party, wrapped in bed sheets, in someone's messy living room. You're the only one of the guests who has your broad, muscular torso exposed. I wonder if this means you are arrogant about your body, if you know how good it is. It makes me wonder how mine will match up.

I look around at the other boys, downing shots and laughing too loud, throwing back their heads. You stand apart with another guy, holding beers, absorbed in a conversation. They seem childlike, babyish compared to you.

I feel your eyes on me but I don't look back: I talk to the friend I've come with. I steal a glance at you and you smile – I think, this can't be real.

I know the friend you're with – he tried to kiss me once at a party, even though he has a girlfriend. I feel myself walk across the room, kiss him on both cheeks.

He introduces me to you, and our eyes lock.

I feel electricity jump between us, hoping I'm not imagining it. Later, I pull up your Facebook page and look at the photo of you, blue-shirted, half-smiling at the camera. I click back through pictures of you laughing in the sun, holding a hammer in front of some construction site. Driving a tractor, muck smeared across your face. I search for clues you might have left, for someone who could be looking.

*

Alone, I walk the cobbled streets, crossing open green spaces, longing for my story to begin. To find the kind of all-consuming love I read about in books, and see in films. I want someone to grasp hold of me and pull me into life, to fill the hole inside myself that I can't fill.

I dress each day with care, always ready for someone to fall for me. To watch me across the quad and think – she's beautiful. I long to be special, different. I am drawn to the pretty girls, the Ugg-booted ones with faux-messy blonde hair and slouchy style, wanting to be like them. I try so hard not to try.

I speak stridently in tutorials, where words come easily. I can hold a room, both reading and addressing it at once. I've always felt at home in front of others, being seen. I long to be chosen by the teacher, marked out. As sentences cascade, kaleidoscoping from my mouth, I feel a rightness I don't find elsewhere and long to feel at all times.

I visit my friend in her golden college in an ancient city. She's a big fish, standing out amongst those too intelligent to trust their own worth. Eyes follow her as she walks across campus in her tiny official netball outfit. Girls see her brightness as betrayal, so she hangs out with boys, a group of puppies she orders about, falling over their feet to do as she commands. When she introduces me, they know me as hers already – I feel warm that she has held me high.

It is like being with a celebrity and I bask in it. Returning to my life I feel deprived.

I am shy and cautious around men though I long to be otherwise. I go on dates with boys I kiss in clubs when drunk, who take my number. We go to nice restaurants and they pay; I kiss them chastely goodnight on my doorstep and close the door on them.

I wonder why I don't invite them in. I enjoy the glow of being watched by candlelight, of talking animatedly, of sudden visibility. The catalogue of individual men I kiss seems unimportant, secondary to how I feel when with them. I watch them talk about themselves, asking the right questions, seeing them open up, and think – this is too easy. I am good at making them fall for me, and once they have it seems there is nowhere else to go.

The thought of them taking off my clothes is something else entirely. When I'm alone in my room touching myself, I want them inside me. I imagine sitting on top of them, losing myself in the deep soft moment. But when they are there, holding my hand as we walk down dark streets, I feel weary at the thought, defiant, like a child pushing out her lip and saying no. Being wanted is more important than the wanting itself, which seems superfluous.

Perhaps I am afraid of losing control, of missing a step in my calculated dance.

*

On St Patrick's Day, green clovers on our cheeks, I stand near you with my friends, stealing glances. I long to be bold enough to kiss you, but the most I can do is make eye contact and smile. You catch my drift, moving closer, and I feel the heat of your presence, the power of drawing you closer. You try to kiss me; at first I decline, pleading friendly loyalty, but of course give in. We're swept away, kissing all night, deafening ourselves against a speaker. My hands slip underneath your shirt, my nails digging into your skin. I feel a pulse between my legs.

You walk me home. It begins to snow, which seems a miracle in March, and we are inside a scene from a cheesy movie. I am aware as I smile wide, throwing my head back to laugh at your jokes, of setting a bear trap around your leg, without you noticing.

We take turns to choose our dates. The cinema, we determine too ordinary.

You take me to a skating rink where I glide unsteadily, mocked by youths who ask, 'D'ya need a hand?' You laugh with me, showing off your own skills, moving easily across the ice.

You place your hand on the small of my back and I relish the heat of it. I touch your chest to steady myself and feel the tautness of muscle, allowing myself an imagining of what's underneath your t-shirt. I blink at you and smile.

We catch the bus to the seaside. It is the first warm

day and I wear a mini skirt. You put your hands under it and I feel a thrill, caring about watching eyes though unsure why. We buy fish and chips and eat them on a windy wall, delighting in soft vinegary heat. The wind whips my hair, and you smooth it behind my ears, hold my face in your hands, plant a salty kiss. I feel your tongue in my mouth and think – this is really happening.

We go to the zoo. You buy the tickets, bending towards the glass window. I watch the girl behind it push her chest infinitesimally forward, smile. You smile back, then return to me.

We wander through the families, heavy with pushchairs, following the slow-moving waddle of toddlers. I let myself picture us, one day, family in tow. A girl astride your shoulders, a baby on my hip. I feel a strange shame for thinking far ahead, as if I'm playing a game of chess with someone who doesn't know the board exists. Is that really what I want? I daren't truly ask myself.

I'm torn between this long-term thinking and my short-fuse desire for you, both of which feel wrong, like something I should smother. You reach your arms out to lean against the bars of an enclosure and I watch the muscles flex, surprising myself with a flush of want.

We watch the penguins move in sad, warm circles, the tigers prowling. I take pictures, marvelling at the baby elephant, but you stand back, seem low. I don't like to ask, think perhaps I've done something wrong.

In the gift shop, we buy animals for each other: a lion for you, a zebra for me. Unintentionally, I am prey to your predator.

On the way home, I crack and ask if you're okay.

'It's just not a life,' you say, and I wonder what you mean. The families at the zoo? Us?

'The animals,' you say. 'They should be free.'

I feel bad: it hadn't crossed my mind. Or if it had, I'd thought it was just the way things were, so we could learn, take pictures, have a nice day out.

I take your hand. You look at me and smile.

One night, after we've been dancing with our friends, we walk home together.

We stop to talk on a bench outside my flat and kiss and kiss. I want to climb on top of you, to bite into you like ripe fruit and see how it tastes. I want everyone to see us here.

'Shall we go inside?' I say, breaking away from you. We both know what will happen if we do.

There is a long pause before you say, 'Not yet.'

'Why not?'

'This feels like more than that,' you say. 'Let's wait.'

You're supposed to be the one who's ready, not the other way around. I feel rotten inside and move away, the moment broken, and we say goodnight.

I convince myself I've gone too far, shown a filthy side of me that has repelled you. I've tipped from Madonna into whore and kick myself inside for getting carried away. I talk to friends who admit it doesn't seem like a good sign. If he liked me enough, surely he'd want to sleep with me? What have I done wrong?

You cook pizza. The uneven base belies homemade; I am impressed and say so. The dough is soft and the tomato sauce tangs. As I praise you, your face doesn't change; you look me in the eyes as if untrusting. There is no flash of joy and I wonder why, but don't yet understand.

We sit on the sofa in your shared living room, surrounded by gym weights, the distended wires from an overused play console. The carpet crunches underfoot. There are no curtains at the wide bay windows, looking out on rows of similar stone. A poster on the wall for a film I don't recognise – the outline of a man with a gun – I ask you, making conversation, but you just shrug. It's hard to piece you together from this room of collaboration.

I think of my room: how I arranged it with someone like you in mind. The pouting face of Marilyn Monroe, hair mussed, wrapped in bed sheets, hangs above my bed. The fairy lights, the careful piles of books.

You move close, pulling me towards you – we kiss, and again I feel myself begin to melt. I climb on top of you and you press my hips down; the glow spreads through my body and I want more, but stop: acting on this rising feeling last time made you turn away. I climb off, tell you I should be going.

'Stay the night,' you say. 'There's no one here.'

I shake my head, though inside I say yes.

'I should go,' I say again.

The heat in your eyes dims.

'Okay,' you say.

And then I leave, a lingering kiss before I go.

Walking home, I wonder if I've played things right. In the buffet of girls at university, will holding out achieve anything, except losing your attention? Throwing you to the other girls, who take off their bras and put fingers inside themselves, who act like those on screen.

A mutual friend's birthday party in a dim-lit bar with cavernous corridors where it is easy to lose your way. You find me, we go to buy drinks. You kiss me and I wonder who is watching. Walking up the stairs, you stop, turn us to a full-length mirror halfway up and make me look at us. You – standing tall, smart in a rare suit. Me in a bright blue dress, blonde hair coiled atop my head.

'We look good together,' you say.

I nod, but something feels wrong – like surface is all we have. I need to prove it's not the case, but don't speak these words out loud.

Your friend takes a photo of us that night – looking in each other's eyes, laughing. When I see it, I feel validated, as if the rush I feel from you is visible, evidenced, marked on your face like a tattoo.

We walk home and you ask questions, about my family and who I was before you. I hear my words as I say them, like an echo on a phone line, eerie and unsettling. Am I enough? A strange thrill thunders through me with the not-knowing.

It's the same feeling I had with her, as if I'm playing some sort of game, and want to get to the next level without you noticing.

I'm learning that you're different. You're serious and sensible, think deeply about things. There's something strong about you – something adult, experienced. On the way to a date you've organised you pull a hand-drawn map out of your pocket, prepared in advance to find the right street for the restaurant, and I feel a thrum – that you have carefully considered the details of this night for me. I feel safe in this knowledge, as if you have shown me something soft by accident.

I think, unbidden, of seeing my father cry after his father died, how he sobbed and held me on their bed and I felt shock, that he had feelings too.

I want to change your life, to be the one to open you up to be the best version of yourself. There is a power in that.

One night when we've known each other a while, we sit in our favourite café late at night and I tell you I want to write. I'm afraid you'll laugh or diminish my ambition, but you don't – you simply nod your head as if there's no reason for this mad bright thing not to happen. I know that I have things to say, although I've written little, and seeing you believe it too makes it shine real.

You tell me you want to travel, to have a life of adventure. I take your hand and squeeze, hoping you'll make room for me, a space. I imagine us out there against the world, living bravely, and wonder if it's possible.

'Let's not let each other forget,' I say. 'That we want a grand life.'

You squeeze my hand back, and nod.

That night we return to your flat, your room. There's just space for a double bed, a wardrobe. You lend me a towel to wash my face, a toothbrush. There is no loo roll in the toilet; the bath looks as though it's never been cleaned. I take my makeup off as if removing a shield, return to the room, heart thumping.

You've set your laptop up on the bed.

'I thought we'd watch a film,' you say.

We wait for it to download from an illegal site. It's one of your favourites, and one I've never seen. I wonder if there's a message contained within to pass along. The opening credits have barely ended when you kiss me, and the rest becomes a blur. We kiss, and I am in my comfort zone – I know I'm good at this. Your hands slip under clothes, and so do mine: soon they're coming off and I'm undone. I push myself against you. We ease together slowly: you are big and

I am inexperienced. I wonder if you are too. Before you, there was only one, and he didn't last long. You move inside, and we are here at last. I feel the pressure mount and then release and we fall back, breathing, together.

Once we are under the covers, lying side by side, you speak.

'When do we make this official?' you ask.

I laugh inside, thinking it already was.

'Whenever you like.'

'How about now?' you say.

Home

2008

In the holidays, you come to visit my family house.

I'm jittery in the car, the new context unsettling. You're waiting outside the train station: it's like seeing a polar bear in Tesco.

I drive us to the park, eager for something to do. We take a path under the trees, leading towards a bridge that crosses the river. I am talking, telling you a childhood story, something stretching its wings inside my chest, spilling out of my mouth. It is a pleasant feeling, an opening-up. I see you watching me, vaguely, as if working out the answer to a problem. It is the same look you get when you look at a landscape, at formations of rocks.

When I finish, there is no reaction. This is unnerving. It makes me want to clap, to dance or sing, to carry on. I stay silent, wait.

'Were you ever bullied as a child?' you ask.

I feel my eyebrows go up. I wonder what you mean. Always, with you, there is a reading between the lines, a deciphering of the simple quiet words into what is happening inside your head. 'No,' I say. 'Why?'

You shrug.

'What do you mean?' I say.

'You can't have been bullied,' you say, as if it's obvious. 'You're just so – open.' Your nose wrinkles, as if you have smelled something bad.

I feel myself flush. I see myself as a bud, closed tight.

We walk on. I wait and you begin to talk. Your voice is quiet but clear; I strain to listen. You tell me about a remote boarding school: rambles in the fells as punishment, sport in the rain, a strict hierarchy.

'My brother went there too,' you say, and stop talking.

'Is he older or younger?'

'Older,' you say. 'Year above me.'

'Must have been nice to have him there too,' I say, thinking of my younger sister, how when teachers got us confused, I felt warm inside.

'Not really,' you say. 'We don't get on.'

The words that flowed easily from your mouth now seem to have dried up. I want more, but it's as if a curtain has come down, and something tells me not to draw it back, not yet.

Instead, I talk about my sister, and brother. I tell you funny stories of when we were younger, easy lore. I talk and you nod and smile, but you are far away. I need to trust you will come back. I'm impatient – it's the same feeling as when I'm reading a good book, and long to know what happens next.

My parents are away, so we have the house to

ourselves. As the gates slide open and we drive up to my family home, you give nothing away.

I give you a tour, talking too much. I show you the kitchen, open plan – a seating area at the end with a view of a balcony and the garden beyond. The games room: the colourful childhood posters, DVDs, the craft cupboard. My parents' sitting room, cosy, for evenings in with takeaways. The Posh Lounge and formal dining room, only used for special occasions.

We make dinner together – chicken fajitas – messing up the spotless kitchen. You proffer easy jobs so you can get on with the real work, opening cupboards to find spices not in the recipe.

I read the back of the packet. 'It says the onions will be ready now.'

You turn them with a spatula. 'They need more colour.'

I busy myself with laying the table, putting on music, overthinking songs that play. I heat the tortilla wraps too early, and have to do it again, hoping you don't notice the mistake, though I'm sure you do.

We eat at the kitchen table. The sun is falling outside the window, tinging the trees with light.

I pour us wine; we drink too much, too quickly. I feel light, and strange, that you are here at all, as if I could blink and all this would disappear.

We are in the Posh Lounge.

I can't remember how we ended up here. Who led

who? Perhaps you asked what is through that door? Or perhaps – I drew you here.

The dark blue sofas, soft and never used. This is a room we keep for best, lighting the pristine fireplace only on Christmas Day.

Family photos, ornaments, adorn the mantlepiece. Thick curtains at patio doors looking out onto stone steps leading to the garden. As a child, I remember hiding there; invisible inside the room, visible outside through glass.

You are kissing me, removing all my clothes in front of the unlit grate.

I feel a burning rush through me and I long for you to hurry up. I want to be in that place: a woodland dark with cracking twigs, shifting underfoot. A moment as rare as spotting deer – one move and off they go. We stay, together, hold.

I imagine someone looking in – what would they think of me?

The next day, my family return. The house, which had seemed large with just the two of us, is full.

When I hear their car on the driveway outside, I feel my heart beat fast. I'm worried they will be too much for you, will undo the work I've done.

In the hallway, I smell my mother's perfume as we lean forwards to hug. My father hugs me too, then stands back, appraises you.

I introduce you and my mother smiles. 'We've heard

so much about you,' she says, and it's the wrong thing, gives away too much. I can't look at you as she pulls you in for a hug. You shake my father's hand.

It's my brother's birthday and we're all here. We open the patio doors and sit in the kitchen, drinking wine while the long evening stretches, lit with fading sun. My mother cooks and we all pronounce it the best meal she's ever made, as we always do. She points out things she'd change, and we shout her down, determined to see only good things. This is a place I feel deeply myself, where the world seems easy, warm and safe.

I act the same as always – bolder, perhaps, than in my normal life. I'm the oldest, and I feel strong here, don't second-guess myself. I know that these people will love me no matter what. I want you to see this bright, clear side of me, to be in awe of it. But with your eyes on me, I question things and wonder why.

They ask you about yourself, about the farm where you grew up. My mum tries to make it easy for you. You answer them, make jokes, and everyone laughs.

Is this going well? I think.

After dinner, we go to the Posh Lounge, and give my brother his birthday presents. We glance at each other, smile a secret smile, thinking what we did in here last night.

We each hand my brother our gifts; he opens them, then hugs and thanks us.

When we go to bed, you seem quiet, drawn. I ask if you're okay.

'You really like each other,' you say, and I blink and say we do.

We walk through our city late at night. The cobbled streets, the tall stone houses, the maze of buildings like some mystic, unsolvable puzzle. You always know the way. We drink in warm, old pubs, sitting by the window, commenting on passers-by. The place is new, exciting, shared.

As summer spreads we know our time is running out. The long holiday looms – we have separate plans away and each moment feels more pressing. We linger in the warmer days, finding sunny spots in large, exposed gardens. We lie together on the grass, talking of nothing and everything, placing our hands on each other's bodies as if warming them after a long, cold winter. I try to preserve these moments in my mind – golden and passing by so fast – how your face is lit for me, and the ease with which our words slip over each other. We open up – a first for both of us – and I'm reminded of feelings I had at school that I was afraid I'd never find again.

As you relax, your stiff exterior softens and you become silly, chasing me around the gardens with a daft grin on your face. I scream and run away, letting you catch me and plant a kiss. You make jokes: you're funny, which I don't expect – each time you drop a dry one-liner is like an unexpected gift and I laugh harder with surprise.

We lie in bed until the early afternoon, talking and touching. I had assumed you would be serious in bed, slow-paced and calm, and sometimes you are, but you also take control, and know what to do.

This – these sunny moments, laughing, feeling beautiful – are how I imagined love. I craved this feeling and now it's here I drink it in.

We try new things: spending hours under the flow of the shower in my shared bathroom until my angry flatmate bangs on the door. I'm inexperienced and want to learn how to touch you with my hands and mouth. My eagerness arouses you: you love it when my desire is authentic, almost automatic. It turns you on to turn me on, which is not something I had learnt from teenage magazines, which were focused on How To Please Your Man.

You tie me up with long black ropes, taking time to wind them around my wrists and ankles. You rub the rough edges along my nipples, and I gasp, throwing my head back and exposing my neck. I feel my eyes roll back as you slowly work your way down my body; I long for your fingers between my legs. When it happens, I feel relief and utterly surrender. I lose track of where we are, of who is winning, of everything. These moments when I'm truly there and not pretending are when you are the most aroused.

*

I meet your parents in a small restaurant on a narrow winding street. I spend time choosing what to wear, settling on a dress and black tights, the skirt just long enough. You wear jeans and a shirt.

'Do you think they'll like me?' I ask on the way there.

'They won't tell you if they do.'

I feel my face collapse, smile slipping. 'What do you mean?'

'My dad will make it hard for you, so be prepared.'

You check for traffic, crossing the road without waiting.

I catch up. 'I'm sure they're lovely.'

You smile tightly, don't reply. It's almost anger on your face, I can't decipher it. I feel a bubble of anxiety rise, push it hurriedly away. We're approaching the restaurant, and there's no going back.

Inside, it's dim – 'romantic' – candlelit – and I search through the gloom, wondering which they are. You see them, jaw stiff, and raise a hand. As we cross the room, your father gets to his feet. He's tall and looks like you, his neck slightly bent forwards as if he's spent a lifetime ducking beams. He smiles, a semi-turn of lips. As you introduce us, I lean in for a hug, feel his stiff body soften fractionally.

Your mother is smiling; she wears a jewel-bright top, brassy hair shining as she moves her head. She has a necklace on of garish beads, and as she stands I see she's small. I hug her too and catch the faintest whiff of cigarettes, feel clear grey eyes appraise me as I sit.

We order wine – she takes the lead – choosing a Pinotage and Chablis too. She tastes when they arrive, and nods her head so everyone else can drink.

'How was your journey up?' I ask.

'Good,' your mother says. 'We've been to see a dog.'

I nod as if this is a normal thing to say.

'My dad has sheepdogs,' you explain, the first time you have spoken. 'Was it a pup?'

'Yes,' your father says. 'The breeder's good. He's trained some winners, so it's looking promising.'

'He does sheepdog trials,' your mum fills in. 'He got to the National one year.'

'Wow,' I say, 'I've never seen a trial.'

'Are you a city girl?'

I smile. 'I thought I was from the countryside, but your son's informed me that I'm not.'

'She's a townie,' you say.

'It's a village.'

'Not London, then, at least,' your father says, a sparkle in his eyes. 'You'll have to come and see the farm.'

'I'd love to,' I say, 'I've heard all about it.'

The waiter comes and takes our order. Your mother orders moules, and I do the same, then worry she'll think I've copied her. Both men order meat.

'We've not heard much about you, dear,' his mother says, pouring out more wine.

I simply smile, not sure what to say. We've been

together months and months; it's tempting to wonder why now? But we're here, and that's enough.

'Never brought a girl home yet,' your father says. 'We wondered if he was gay.'

You look down at the table.

'I better play my cards right then,' I say, and we all laugh, the tension lifting like bubbles in champagne.

As we eat our mains, your father turns to me. 'I hear you like to read.'

'I study English, so you'd hope so,' I say, and your mother smiles.

'Have you read much Thomas Hardy?'

'I've read *Tess*.'

'I like his poetry,' he says, and you nearly spit out your wine.

'Poetry?' you say. 'I didn't think you could read!'

We all laugh.

We say goodbye outside the stone facade, the light of afternoon bright after the dim inside. I hug them both, and say I hope to see them soon.

Your father winks. 'I'm sure you will.'

You roll your eyes, shake your father's hand, and we are off, walking up the hill together.

'How do you think that went?' I say.

'They liked you,' you say, and it's all I need to hear.

You are strange and silent for a few days after your parents' visit.

We go to the Highlands together, driving my tiny

silver car. I put music on, and sing along, as she and I used to when we were teenagers. You don't join in; I turn it down.

We watch the city dissipate and the green land stretch, following the broad roads towards the majesty of the Forth Road Bridge. The hillocks roll upwards until they become dwarfing peaks, as the houses thin out and heather and sheep take precedence. I take photos: you at the wheel, smiling, the mountains that start to reveal themselves.

We drive towards a point you have chosen on a map. It feels good to have direction, purpose, freedom.

You turn up the music, sing tunelessly, and I smile.

We take a winding road through a valley, following the meandering roar of a river. I roll the window down, wanting to hear the water crash over rocks. You pull over to the side of the road.

'This is the spot,' you say.

We pitch the tent – long and blue – just big enough for two. We collect firewood – lumps of dampened wood, fallen arms of trees, bracken and twigs – and build a fire together. You light it, and we sit on waterproof coats, watching the flames as the evening sun fades. We cook steaks and asparagus in a pan you've brought, and drink cans of warm beer, chinking them together.

'Cheers,' you say. 'To us.'

*

The next day, we drive the car to a secluded spot, overlooking the fields below. A craggy outpost, we walk through a rocky valley until we emerge and the land spreads out below us. It gives me vertigo to look down over the cliff-like edge, to think of all those small houses below, of the lives going on within them.

I watch your side profile – jawline, a softness around your eyes – and wonder again what you're thinking but don't ask.

We take a seat close to the edge of the cliffs, hidden by rocks.

You turn to me. 'What is your fantasy?'

I wonder what you mean. 'In life?'

'No. What do you think about when you come?'

I realise you are talking about sex. I think about last night in the tent, you above me. What do I think about when I come? Nothing.

'I don't know.'

'You must know,' you say.

Must I? I feel inadequate, foolish, pressure to find the right words.

'What about when you're alone?' you say.

'I use my vibrator and I come.'

'But what do you think about?'

'Nothing,' I say.

'There must be something.'

I can tell you think I'm holding something back, and I search myself for the answer. I think about those moments, about fantasies, and immediately, I think about her. About those furtive moments when we were younger, and how they've always hovered within me. I don't want to say that aloud.

'Sometimes, I think about other women.'

Your eyebrows rise. 'Really?'

'Yes.'

Looking down, I see that you are hard and feel a mix of pleasure and irritation. I have said the right thing, have elicited a reaction, but it's as if your dick swells to fill all available space. My mind is clouded with your physicality.

I've said something I have never said out loud before, something so deep I wasn't sure there were words for it. I have opened a door only to find it leads to your want and not my own. I'm irritated with you for eclipsing me.

I have a fervent desire to be alone, unpestered. But the moment passes, like the clouds that float above. I look down and see your trousers bulge and that look in your eyes – an animal look – and feel myself shift into autopilot. It's easy to find the words now that you are in that place, to keep you there. I talk of showers, falteringly, of kissing girls at school. The more I see the effect of the words, more words follow.

Where does this lead? We're in a public place.

I could touch you now and take the lead, but don't, frozen by some unnamed voice that says no. Behind some rocks, what would I do, if you put your hand on my leg? If you drew it up towards that darker place. Would I want you to?

You are not bold enough yet and part of me is glad. We wait and descend, towards the other people and the waiting car.

Away

2009

We spend the summer apart, writing long emails – you tell me of your fieldwork, mapping the rocks on some Greek island, of the boys you've gone with, of sunburns and beers, dodgy Greek haircuts, sheltering in a cave to eat your lunch because of a sudden storm.

I write to you of London: days working in a literary agency unpaid, of evenings out in bars with friends, eating morsels of cheese and drinking too much wine.

'I hope there are no men,' you type.

'Maybe there are,' I reply.

I imagine you toned and tanned and beautiful surrounded by rocks and tell you so. You send me a photo and ask for some in return. I spend hours in my room of the shared flat, posing for a camera held aloft, seeing myself anew through the lens: my face lit warm with makeup and dim light, my arms thrust together to lift my breasts.

I choose each image, collating a sample to send across the world.

All day at work I wonder if you've seen them, feeling a pulse of power at you thinking of me, opening them in the internet café. I look over the photos again, reassure myself. I wonder if I would care if you showed your friends, if I would want you to.

You take two days to reply – the café is a walk from where you're staying, and you're busy all day, tired at night. I check my email, tricking myself that I do not care.

When the reply comes, the first line makes my heart race. 'Wow,' you say. 'Your amazing. You've made me want you so much. Send more if you can.'

I forgive the grammatical error and smile inside.

You ask if I had fun taking the photos. I say yes because I know it is the right answer, but fun did not come into it. The thought of being carried away on my own wings feels alien. Collating the photos had felt more like choosing artworks for an exhibition, a left-brained task, designed to impact the viewer, not myself.

The messages we send get longer, more detailed. We tell each other minor details of our days and there is space and time to ask questions. It's easier in some ways – your words fall out of you on the screen. You tell me you're missing me, while having the time of your life. I tell you about a promotion at work, which I joke is moot as I am still unpaid. You root for me and I am happy you are there to share it with.

My friends ask about you and I tell them you are kind and smart and really fit. I feel relief to finally have someone to talk about. It doesn't stop us flirting with other boys in bars, though. I still love the feeling of drawing them towards me, of lighting myself up and watching them want, but I never overstep a line. I wonder if you do, but something tells me you don't. You seem too rational to make a rash decision based on lust.

Returning to university, I look forward to seeing you, wanting to prove to myself you're real. I put on new lingerie and you come round, burying your face in me. These moments, when we're drawn together, tell me everything I need.

My flatmates and I hold a house-warming in the first week of university – it's for my birthday. I'm living with a soft-hearted American girl – you can't understand her, her raw emotions. As she talks, you look at her as if she keeps flashing you her underwear.

My other flatmate is French and beautiful – when we've been out together, we turn heads. We'd dance close, like my best friend and I did at school, and once we kissed for the bouncer to get into a VIP area of our favourite club. I felt powerful as I pulled her towards me, and wondered if it was her first time with another girl. She's fun, but also determined, studying hard, effortlessly running across campus in the early mornings.

When the house is full and thronging, music filling my mind, I lose track of you, greeting friends I haven't seen all summer. When I find you, you're talking to the American, and your face is difficult to read.

She's leaning in – has had too much to drink. As I approach, her face softens; she moves one step away.

'Sorry,' I say. 'There's too many people.' *I'm popular* is what I'm really trying to say.

'He's been fending for himself,' the American says.

'I'm fine,' you say. 'Don't feel you need to babysit me.'

'I don't,' I say. 'I wanted to see you.'

You look beyond me, at the door. 'I'm going to go. I've got an early lecture.'

'Oh, okay.'

'I'll call you in the morning.' You lean in to kiss me, on the cheek. 'Have fun.'

We watch you leave, and then I turn to her.

'That was strange,' I say. 'What were you talking about?'

She looks at her nails. 'I was teasing him.'

'What do you mean?'

'Just letting him know how precious you are.'

I'm confused; I want to follow you, to make you talk to me.

'Let's get some drinks,' she says. 'You don't need him to have fun.'

She's right: we do shots in the kitchen then head out, dancing all night. We frequent the smoking area and I smoke out of spite – you hate it because of your mother. I flirt with your friend, ask where you are, acting as if I don't care, don't know you've gone home. 'Not sure,' he says, 'I thought he was with you tonight.'

The music's good and all my friends are here. I tell

myself I don't miss you at all, looking around at all the faces, feeling love.

It's only in the morning, waking alone and late, that I feel wrong. I check my phone – no message.

I go out to lectures, losing myself in books. I speak boldly in my tutorial, holding court, as if to prove I'm strong. When I check my phone, I have a message from you – *Can we talk?* And I reply – *Of course. Do you want to come round?*

So you do. I open the door to the flat; we hug, then go to my bedroom.

Your face is closed.

'What's wrong?' I say.

'Things feel different,' you say. 'Since we came back. Don't you think so?'

'We've only been back a few days.'

'I know.'

And then there's nothing else. Just silence and a scream inside my head. How can this be happening? I think of all those summer messages sent, of you, leaning over me, eyes locked, the feelings there, just two days ago.

'What do you want to do?' I say.

'Break up.'

I feel the sickness in my stomach twist. I can't think of what to say. Do I submit? Or try to convince you that you're wrong, that we've got something good? It feels too desperate so I don't.

'Okay,' I say.

You look relieved that there will be no battle, and then you say, 'Perhaps we can be friends.'

I feel as if you've slapped me. 'What would be the point of that?' I'm sharper than I mean to be, and your face looks shocked.

'Because I like you,' you say.

No you don't, I think.

'I can't be friends with you. If we bump into each other, I'll be nice, but I can't promise more than that.'

'Okay,' you say, and you look genuinely sad.

You can't have it all, I think.

'I'm going to go,' you say.

I nod, and then I hear the front door click shut.

I lean back against the wall. This can't be real. All those building blocks we've placed so carefully, all those collated moments, all come tumbling down.

I go into the kitchen where my flatmates are making tea. They look up as I come in.

'He just broke up with me,' I say.

'What?' the French girl says. 'That makes no sense.'

Her outrage mirrors mine and I am glad. 'I know.' I turn to the American. 'What exactly did you say to him last night?'

She shrugs. 'Just how awesome you are. How much we love you.'

'It doesn't seem enough.'

'Maybe he'd been having doubts before? Did something happen in Greece?'

I think back to the stream of messages, the pictures,

his words in black and white. 'I don't think so,' I say. 'We've been writing to each other all summer.'

They look at me and I feel foolish and humiliated. All those things I said, pulled away.

'Well, at least we're all single now,' she says.

It feels as if I've been training for a marathon and then broken my leg the day before the race.

It's hard. I walk through campus with headphones in, skipping love songs.

I wrestle inside, telling myself I am enough, I'm special. That I don't need you.

I dress up for nights out, leaning close to the mirror and trying to really see myself, to cover up whatever flaw I have that made you leave. I am determined not to repeat the same mistake, to be better next time. It makes me feel so tired that I'll need to start again, with someone new.

I go over and over in my head moments we've shared, replaying them differently. They felt right, but they weren't.

I write about it, this feeling. Trying to puzzle out where things went wrong on paper. I'm not sure how I feel until I read the words back.

I think of all the things I want to do, all the things I will one day be.

I try to think of all the things I already am, but none of it feels enough.

*

My parents come to visit. We go to the Indian restaurant as planned, changing the reservation to three.

They come to my flat first; my mother is dressed up, smells of home. She hugs me, then snoops around. I let her, showing her each room – my bedroom with a large bed and window looking out onto the street, the living room with a broad bay window, and the rooms of the other two.

'It's nice,' she says.

My father stands by, rocking on his heels.

I turn to them.

'If we bump into him, you are to say nothing,' I say.

They glance at each other and nod.

Luckily, we don't cross paths and make it to the restaurant safely. Although this Indian restaurant is different from the one we go to in my hometown, there is a familiarity to the menu – we often go out for Indian at home. I look across the table at my parents and they seem soft-edged with nostalgia.

'Thanks for coming,' I say.

My mother reaches for my hands. 'How are you?' she says, her eyes all concern.

'I'm fine,' I say. 'Really.'

'He's a fool,' my father says, too loudly, and the feeling in his words is like a balm.

My best friend and I meet at the airport, run into each other's arms as if it's been years not weeks. The last time – in a pub in our hometown – I was still with you.

We smoked too many cigarettes and danced all night, shielded by our respective men. Now, I feel exposed, defeated; I smell her hair, don't want to let go.

'Are you okay?' she says. 'You sounded strange on the phone.'

'I'm fine.'

'You're doing that thing, where you pretend everything's fine, even when it's not.'

'No, really. It's his loss.'

She just looks at me. 'We'll talk about it later.'

On the flight to Prague, we order drinks and buy cigarettes from duty-free. We look through photos on our phones, of summer nights when everything was good.

We have an apartment on a seedy road, opposite the dark swirl of the river, but not in the picturesque part of town. We're surrounded by bars with pictures of bikini-clad women outside, flickering lights and views into dank basements. The flat has a small kitchen and a bedroom; paint peels from the walls, stock images remain in cheap, fake-wood frames.

It's cold and we are unprepared. We head out into the streets, arm in arm, our heads bent into the wind. Near the castle we buy fur hats and take photos in a little garden, a small patch of green in the austere grandness of the city. She takes red lipstick out of her pocket and holds my face up to the light, applying it. We hold the camera aloft and pout into the lens, mocking but not-mocking ourselves.

We find a café in a side street near the main square and order Irish coffees to warm up. She tells me how she learnt to pour the cream for these, working in a restaurant at university. I feel a stab of jealousy that our lives have continued without each other, that there are so many new things she's done without me. She has a university best friend – so do I – and we try not to mention them. I imagine them together, laughing, and it hurts.

She lights a cigarette, inhales, lights mine too.

'So,' she says.

I knew this moment would come, but not so soon – we've only just arrived.

I think about saying I'm fine.

'I'm in denial,' I say and she nods. 'I miss him. I'm mourning what we could have had. And there's nothing I can do.'

I don't want to but I cry.

She wipes my cheeks. 'I don't understand,' she says, shaking her head. 'Is he an idiot?'

I smile. 'He's not. That's what makes it worse. He's sensible, makes good decisions. I did everything right. I'm just not enough.'

'You are,' she says.

'Maybe I'm meant to be alone,' I say.

'You're not,' she says. 'But what's so wrong with that?'

'I want someone else to see it too,' I say. 'To see me. He did, and walked away. I can't deny that's true.'

She takes both my hands. 'I see you. And I always will.'

Because it's her, I believe it.

We make our way around the square, drinking vodka, which we feel is the national drink, though we don't bother to check. I'm glad we came, grateful that I have her and she has me. She's right – she's seen me all along, at worst and best, and she's still here.

We reapply our red lipstick periodically and it acts like a shield, a costume for the people we are in Prague. We eat dumpling stew in a bistro by the river, drink beer and smile at local boys. Suddenly, it is 2am and we're dancing with a stag do, showing them how fun their wives used to be. They are like zoo animals, escaped for just one night. I kiss one of them up against a wall outside the club, thrilled to be moving further away from you. His mouth is smaller and he's a bad kisser, but I pretend he's not.

She and I share a single bed though there are two in our room.

Two weeks later I cook lunch for a friend from school who's on your course – my go-to dish of salad with ravioli and mozzarella.

'Have you heard from him?' she asks.

'No,' I say. 'I deleted his number.' I hate the pride in my voice.

'What would you do if he got back in touch?'

I feel the walls rebuild. 'I wouldn't be able to trust him again.'

She looks at me.

'What?' I say.

'I saw him on the bus just now,' she says. 'He seemed sad. He was staring out of the window. I asked him what was wrong and he said it's you.'

Against my will, my heart jumps. 'I don't know what to say.'

'Perhaps he'll message you.'

I shrug and turn back to the pasta.

That night, my phone buzzes.

It looks like a random number, but it's you.

A long message, carefully written, without any spelling errors. You ask if I will meet.

I'm tempted to write back *Who is this?* but don't.

Okay. Our place, tomorrow night at 8.

I feel sick all day, even more so on the way there, deliberately five minutes late. I can't bear the thought of sitting waiting for you. Carefully getting ready, I resolve to be firm.

You're there, sitting in our usual booth. I've spent the past few weeks convincing myself that you don't exist, and now there you are. You glance up and I think of your father: the wariness of your gaze, as if you don't trust the ground beneath your feet.

You get up; we hug. I hold my breath, but still your smell is there.

'Do you want a drink?' you ask.

'Just water, thanks.' You have a pint of beer.

You go to order, sit back down.

'Thanks for coming,' you say. 'You look nice.'

I keep my face still. 'What did you want to say?'

'I think I've made a mistake.'

I don't say anything.

'I got scared.'

'What does that mean?'

'The party. All your friends. I looked around and felt this great responsibility. That my actions could hurt you.'

'Your actions have hurt me.'

You look upset. 'I'm sorry. I didn't know what else to do.'

'Maybe talk to me about it? Don't just flee.'

'I'm sorry.'

'Stop saying that.'

'Can we try again?'

'What's made you change your mind?'

'I've missed you.'

I think of photos placed on social media to show you I didn't care. I wonder if they've worked. I want to tell you how I saw you across a club one night, dancing with your friends, laughing. How it stung.

You're waiting for an answer.

'How do I know you won't do this again?'

You look right at me. 'I won't.'

I imagine saying no, walking out of here. I think of returning to lonely walks, to longing. I look at you, watching me. I see you turn your head, sip your drink. This doesn't feel over.

'We'll have to take things slow. Go back to dates again. I'm not promising anything.'

You take my hand and smile, as if you've won.

I try to make it hard for you, to make myself a prize that needs winning. Although I miss your body, the closeness of your skin, I feel I should keep you at arm's length. Denying you access makes me feel in control, is a way of testing your true feelings. Do you really want *me*, or just what's underneath my clothes?

You invite me for a massage night, and though I know I should say no, I say yes. I feel weak at opening the doors to myself so easily, but do it anyway. I want to be back in that place, on the open road with you, seeing where we go. This is how much I need to see myself through your eyes. I wonder why my own view of myself is not enough. I push the thought away.

When I arrive, you've laid towels on the bed, bought special oil, lit candles, and this is new and different. I let my eyes close, let myself enjoy the way your hands move. You have this way of knowing what to do, where to go next, how to build tension. I am biting my lip, arching my back, clenching my fists. My body calls for you, overcoming the sound of my thoughts, which have been deafening these last few weeks.

Afterwards, we lie together, and you look into my eyes. I can see there is real affection there, the beginnings of love maybe. But I can also see your fear. Between us there's a tussle which goes unspoken.

On the way home, I walk through dark streets and I begin to cry. I feel all the emotions I've held back rush forward now that I am safe, and don't need to be brave. It feels foolish now that some resolution has been found, but I allow it.

You take me to the Highlands again – driving us higher and higher through snow-covered peaks. We pass a herd of deer, grazing on the side of the road, and you pull the car over. I watch their shadowy figures move slowly through the flurrying snow and think of the first night we walked home together.

You keep stealing glances at me; I don't let myself look back. I hold myself still inside this moment, sensing something is changing between us, stretching out. I'm not breathing, not moving, as if I'm out there in the cold wind amongst the deer and don't want to frighten them away. Everything inside me wants to grab hold of you and shake.

A few times, you open your mouth, but no words come out.

'I love you,' you say, finally.

I hear a gasp escape me, and then I say it back.

When we get back to the accommodation, we light the wood-burning stove and make dinner: it feels as if we're homemaking. I feel a roaring joy that this is happening. We make jokes and laugh lightly. Your smile is broad and bright across the table.

After dinner, we fall onto the bed. We've brought

my camcorder and I pull it out of my suitcase, switching it on, seeing you reflected in the tiny screen. We talk and laugh and I hear our voices more heavily.

You take the camera from my hands and hold it up, pulling me gently onto the bed and kissing me. I'm aware of you capturing us on tape, of preserving this moment. We are here, and also in that small square of light. We are being watched, seen. As I take off my clothes, I imagine us playing this tape one day, and remembering how close we were, how safe inside this moment, together. It feels like a timelapse film of a flower, opening up.

When we're both naked, you hold the camera while I go down on you. I see myself: the slut, the whore, the sort of girl who does wild things. Is that what you want from me? Is it what I want for myself?

When we fuck, the camera stays, but I long to be just with you, to be inside what is happening rather than observing it. After a while, I push the camera away and pull you close, kissing you, holding on to the sides of your face until you forget the lens too. I try to give myself to you, to this moment, but there's still a small tender part of me I hold back.

Next Level

2009

A stone farmhouse, sitting astride a hill, visible from the long, untarmacked drive. Inside, an Aga, a huge dresser, two windows looking out over the valley.

The room is empty: the smell of cigarette smoke and a steaming cup of black coffee. The silence is intense, heavy.

We walk together, trudging in wellies across the wet land. We stop, looking out over fields of varying green, dark patches of woodland and forest like unkempt pubic hair. You put your arms around me from behind.

Your lips find mine, as if searching for something, wanting something from me. I turn, but you don't let me, sliding your hand inside my jeans, under your mother's coat, inside me. I try to pull your hand away – it's daylight, anyone could see – but then there is a feeling between my legs, spread like honey on buttered toast, and I move myself apart. With your other hand you grasp my breast then pull down my trousers.

The chill of wind, you bend me forward – the view is beautiful and I feel you inside, pressing deep as you move in and out. I watch the trees ahead of us, cresting the edge of the hill, outlined with green moss as if lit from below.

I imagine you here.

Running through the fields, tinkering in the disused barns. You've told me stories of shooting rabbits, of running free. The youngest child of four: an afterthought, always overlooked, one step behind your older, bolder siblings.

Your brother took the spotlight and held it over himself, protective of it, pushing you to one side, making sure you never questioned the way things were supposed to be. He is the last of your family I meet. He's charming, smiling broadly, pulling me in for a hug. Fox-like, he's a less good-looking version of you with a sharper, wily face. He says and does everything right, but I know too much about him already. I know how he called you fat and stupid and made you sad and closed inside. I hate him for it, but also wonder if you're how you are – kind, thoughtful, caring – because you didn't want to be like him.

Your mother is strong: brittle and sharp, she drinks too much and says exactly what she thinks. I admire her brightness, even after all these years, and we get on. I can see she has been hurt too many times. I can also see how much she loves you, even if she can't say it aloud.

Your father is the thump on the ceiling, the creak of a floorboard, the splosh of water heard from a long drawn bath. I feel him everywhere, but he rarely speaks. You hate it when people say you look alike. You tell me you have few memories of him as a child, except for a trip to the city once, ice creams in a park, when some test results made him believe he was dying.

Coming here, I see you in chinks, pieces that come together slowly like a developing photograph. I long for more but cannot ask.

We return to university. I feel privy to some special knowledge about you, seeing you anew against the old stone buildings as we walk side by side.

She comes to visit, arriving on the train. I go to collect her, waiting on the platform until I spot her confident swinging walk, her height, the heads that turn in her direction.

We go to a pub near the station and catch up. She's had an argument with her boyfriend – he didn't want her going out, and she did it anyway. She has a habit of choosing the most unavailable boy, making them fall in love with her. As soon as this is achieved, their dependence irritates her, and she pushes them away. The harder she pushes, the more pathetic they become.

'He can't tell me what to do,' she says.

'Did you tell him that?'

'Yes. He punched a hole in my wall.'

'What will you do?' I ask.

She shrugs. 'He's sorry now.'

I try to imagine you punching a hole in a wall.

'How's things?' she asks.

'Good. Things feel different,' I say. 'He said he loves me.'

Her hand goes up to her mouth. 'That's huge,' she says. 'Did you say it back?'

'I did,' I say. 'I do.'

You come round to the flat to meet her. You're quiet, and it feels a big effort for you to smile at her. I wonder if you're nervous. She hugs you, makes it easy, goes to fix us drinks.

'What do you fancy? I'm great at negronis.'

'Perfect,' you say.

'She's really into cocktails,' I say, as we follow her to the narrow kitchen. 'It's convenient.'

I watch you make small talk. These two titans of my life in the same room feels almost like a bad omen. She's talking fast, filling silences, and you are listening, nodding. I feel grateful to you both for trying, but also strangely powerful: I am the reason you are making the effort, making yourselves uncomfortable. I am the reason you are both here, in this room now, at all.

As winter turns to spring, the end of university looms and questions of what happens next begin to surface. I walk the streets late at night, luxuriating in having the city to myself, soaking in the last of limbo time, when all future options are still open.

When people ask what I want to do, I say I want to write.

They ask what I have written and I say: nothing.

What I mean is – I have written nothing of substance, nothing complete, nothing you would call writing. I have always written: diaries, thoughts, feelings. Garbled paragraphs about you, about her, part of me relieved to have something to write about. None of it feels serious enough to talk about.

But I know I will do it properly. I know I will show my work, and how scary that might be. I start to think about how.

She and I discuss London – the flat we've always talked about. She has a graduate job working for an alcohol company, after a series of gruelling, terrifying interviews, where inevitably she's shone. There are courses I can take there – one with a famous poet with a brooding stare. I imagine him reading my work, speaking of it, and I apply.

One night, while we work together in our café, I ask you what you'll do. In my mind, I've imagined you might choose London too. After all, where else is there?

You tell me you've applied for jobs – Australia and Africa are on your list.

'I have an interview next week,' you say.

Momentarily, I'm shocked – how have we not discussed this before? I've been wary – so perhaps have you – of doing anything to unsettle the happy equilibrium we've found, but now's the time, it seems, to have this conversation.

I message you good luck on the big day — you call me afterwards.

'I think it went well. They gave me something to solve — I think I got it right.'

That means you did. 'When will you find out?'

'Soon, they said.'

I feign excitement for you, and feel it too, but a low-level anxiety churns. Our paths might diverge at this point, just when things seem steady. Perhaps you will be an episode I talk about in years to come — the university boyfriend — but not a final resting place.

I have an interview too — with the poet. I float down on the train, feeling the world spread out before me as I walk through the city, passing landmarks I know from the Monopoly board. How must it feel to live here, for all of this to be normal? It's as if I'm looking through a gate into a garden but can't find the latch.

There are more people than I thought waiting to be interviewed, and my nerves jangle.

'I liked your piece,' the poet says, when I sit down.

I'd submitted two, and don't like to ask which one.

'It has potential,' he says, and my heart sings. 'But there's lots of work to do. If you get on the course, it will be hard.'

I nod, wondering what he means exactly. I am hungry

to do whatever it takes. I am good at filling other people's expectations, and am desperate to find a way to unlock his.

'Why do you want to write?' he asks.

This question – like asking why I want to walk, or stretch my legs, or fly. What answer does he want to hear? 'I want to make a living from something I love,' I say.

'It's not easy, to make a living from writing,' he says.

Encouraging, I think. 'I want to try. I want to improve, and learn. I want to see how good I can be.'

I want to see my name in lights, I think, but do not say.

'Well, we'll let you know.'

'I loved your book on Keats,' I say and he glances up at me. 'He's my favourite poet.'

He smiles, slightly. 'Thank you. You can go.'

On the train home, I fear I haven't done enough.

Your letter arrives before mine and we celebrate. You'll be leaving after graduation, your path solid and clear. On the other side of the world.

I tell myself to shrug, that we are young and can overcome anything. What will be will be. I want us to be good enough to surpass any challenge, and I let myself believe we are, cultivating the persona of someone I wish I was now.

But what will I do if I am left adrift?

When my letter comes, the envelope is thin – this is a bad sign. I sit on my bed with trembling hands and watch the letter open. Inside, I have been accepted.

I jump up and call my parents, you and her, and all are thrilled.

The day before you leave we drive to Blackpool and walk along the grey beach in driving wind and rain. We eat popcorn and candy floss, walk amongst deserted, rusting rides. We joke that I'm showing you the worst of England so you won't miss it when you're gone. We watch *Australia* the film and I resent red earth and wide open spaces for drawing you away.

I take you to the airport, kiss you goodbye and wish you a safe flight.

'Call me when you land,' I say.

You promise to and kiss me again.

'Are you nervous?' I ask.

'No,' you say, but I think you are – a little. So many things unknown, how could you not be? Something drives you far away, some inner desire to prove yourself, away from the small, closeted place you grew up, in the big wide world. I try to understand and let you go.

I drive out of the airport, following signs, turning left and right through roads that uncoil like intestines. I grew up near here and know where to stop – a lay-by near the prison – where I cry, feeling foolish and dramatic. I cry in case this is the end, in case we're not strong enough to find each other again.

I imagine you: an Australian wife and tanned surfer kids – a sunny life beyond my comprehension.

You're in the air for hours: I picture you smiling at the hostess, eating free nuts and drinking beer. I see you sleeping, mouth ajar, and want to smooth your brow, to take photos and laugh when you wake up. You're all alone out there and when you call, I'm glad.

'Is it sunny?' I ask.

'Of course. It's the middle of the afternoon. And there?'

'It's raining and it's dark.'

'Of course it is.'

'Do you miss it already?'

'I miss you.'

'Go on, make a life for yourself. I'll speak to you tomorrow.'

Solo

2009

A shiny black door, chipped paint – unnoticeable in a row of shops like a door to another world.

She's there when I arrive, parking my car illegally on Fulham High Street. She's chosen the flat for us, sent me photographs – it's strange to be inside it looking at the boxes, labelled in her spiky handwriting. She's started to unpack: books on a tea-ringed coffee table, cushions on the sagging sofa, a string of fairy lights upon the mantlepiece. Finally, we're here – living together in the big city.

'I wanted to make it homely before you arrived,' she says, seeing where my gaze lands.

I pull her towards me, hug her, feel our heartbeats together again.

'It's finally happening,' I say.

'I know,' she says.

We put on loud music, jump around as we unpack. Her father has given her a bottle of champagne and we open it warm, the cork ricocheting from the ceiling, making us laugh, leaving no trace. As we unpack our clothes into wardrobes that barely open in too-small rooms, we show each other – remember this, you wore that when – and try things on, parading up and down the hallway.

We pull open the sash window in the living room and smoke. London creeps into the room: far-away sirens, the dull roar of traffic, the sound of children laughing. We can smell curry from the Indian restaurant downstairs.

That night we dress up, doing each other's makeup as we did when we were seventeen. We're adults now, we think. We're free.

Heels clatter on cobbles as we walk the narrow path towards the Tube station.

Before we know it, we're on the platform, snapping photos on a bench.

Ordering shots at some sleek new bar, we're almost wild with dreams come true. How many times have we imagined this – being far away alone together, taking on the world? Now it's here, and we smile wide, and there's nowhere in the world I'd rather be.

My tutor has the face of an author photo – deep lines, bushy brows, downturned lips, eyes that express displeasure. A face designed to catch the light, shadowed like a charcoal drawing.

He is often silent, making me hold my breath, lightheaded at the thought he'll glance at me, or look deeper and find me wanting. Which of us around this table has what it takes? Does he have a way of knowing? Or the power to make it so?

His words are given frugally, made currency by supply and demand. I long for them, feeling the deepness in my body.

Over weeks we practise giving feedback as the spotlight rolls around. My turn – I can't look at anyone, as if I've performed surgery on myself and am left open on the table, heart visibly beating while they circle overhead. Any good words are pocketed. I learn to hear the questions, finding answers later when alone. I nod, write notes, trusting that I will know what to do.

I walk the streets near the flat, stopping in coffee shops. Opening documents, staring at words, trying to tease out the best ones. I need to crack the glass, break through, but don't know how. Their voices are too loud. It's a relief to listen to them, rather than pausing, listening for my own.

She watches me, sitting beside me at copper-burnished bars. In her light, I shine.

I talk to men, despite you. I draw them in with words and looks. Mainly, I listen. I know it is the way to make them want me, to hold up a mirror that reflects their best light back.

'You're good at this,' she says, impressed.

I shrug it off, but know I am.

'It's a shame you're not single,' she says. 'You'd have some fun.'

I wonder about this, about what freedom would mean. But I know I am bold partly because you're there, behind me, even from the other side of the world, bolstering, holding me up. I have nothing to lose, so gamble easily.

Slowly, something forms; the beginning of a novel, perhaps.

The feeling of words rolling out of me is intoxicating and makes me come alive.

I look at them, after, and try to shift them into how they feel inside. I try to reflect, in words, my inner world. But when I return to them, it's like looking at my face in a magnifying mirror. The words distort, will not comply.

Sometimes I lie awake and fear there's nothing there – that I won't be good enough to make it work. What then? I'll get an ordinary job and accept an ordinary life. I hope it doesn't come to that – the thought drives me forward.

In the evenings, she and I frequent the pub across the road. She talks of work – an office, so grown-up! – and all the things she does to make the business work. She's in marketing and gets invited out – we go to parties and drink free and feel we're living the life we've always wanted.

We hold parties too, cramming people in, dancing on a coffee table we found on the side of the road. We stay out all night – with no one to call us home, why not? We drink too much and fish for men, though we are unavailable. There are no rules and I am glad, sometimes, you are not here.

In many ways, my life is easier without you – I have space to find my thoughts, to write. To truly, safely be myself.

I cut my hair and dye it dark without the fear that you won't like it.

We stretch our wings, and it feels good, to be both cared for and be free. We simultaneously pursue our dreams, running on parallel lines across the world.

We speak each day on Skype, learn new ways to be intimate, making noises to a camera, watching each other come in pixels on a screen.

We brighten each other's day – a relationship between the hours when we're both awake.

New World

2010

All things thrown into sharp relief.

The light dazzles, sliding off everything, bleaching the curtains, relentlessly crystal clear. It sinks to golden red as the sun melts, slipping below the horizon like honey swallowed. The trees are darker green, lush with broad, speckled white trunks. I press my hands against them and the outer bark peels away.

The earth – it feels wrong to call it soil – is red and has a deepness, a dryness. Scrub grasses try to grow and fail.

The sea is a marvel, the waves crashing, curving, hiding dangerous things.

All that is solid, real, dissolves into air. This place has existed, all along, on the other side of the world. While we sit here, sipping our coffee, my mother and father are sleeping, turning in bed, waking, washing, shitting. My friends ride the Tube, rattling underground to familiar places, and we are far away.

I fly through a day to reach you.

After passport control I find a toilet, change clothes,

spray perfume. I wash my face, splashing away the muggy sky with cold water. I apply makeup, hoping your memories of me haven't dulled the reality, that I won't be a disappointment.

You are waiting in Arrivals. I see you before you see me – your eyes scan the crowds, unsmiling.

You see me and smile.

I smile back.

I'd wondered if I'd run towards you, throw myself into your arms. I long to be confident enough to do so. I walk and we embrace. You look tanned, your face relaxed. Your broad arms and chest are mine again.

You wheel my suitcase outside, where the heat is startling, everything bright and clean, as if a new world has been conjured just for us. We find your small gold car and climb in, pulling out of the airport onto a broad highway.

I first see the city across the river, the glistening blue glass skyscrapers lined up like a mirage. I can't wait to walk amongst them, looking up and feeling small.

We talk of the journey, the films I've watched. I feel the magnetism of your wanting, and fizz with happiness and anticipation – know I must live up to it. You are here again and magnify to fill the space; it is both a relief and a disappointment not to be the centre of things again. Perhaps making you happy is easier than making myself happy.

We park under your building and climb in a lift to the ninth floor. Your apartment is bigger than it seemed on screen and it's strange to be here – in real life – to touch the sofa, where you sit, to see your laptop on the table.

We drink a beer and then you kiss me. Our clothes come off, remembering how – your body is familiar and your taste, the way you touch me. All those stalled moments online were marathon foreplay – waiting to be here. I pull you into me, wanting you to feel the moment as I do.

I think of all the other men in bars, how I drew them close, but never crossed an unspoken line.

Soon you are inside and I breathe fast, relieved to find you again. As if all this time, I have been holding my breath – and now exhale at last. You are able to take me out of myself, to make me forget that I exist at all. The crushing pressure of all the things I want to be is lightened as you hold me down: I feel my grip on myself release under yours.

As I slip away below the surface of us, I think of the crashing roar of the waves, deafening and inevitable. I imagine myself floating in the intermittent calm. I long for the sudden pull of the water, to lose my senses in the flow of being under with you.

I have missed how you can do this to me. This place between us that is an escape from myself.

The mesmerising sweet shop where they twist the sugar, folding it over and over until thin, breaking it into tiny candies with small hammers. The city centre – so ordered it skirts dull – the river, moving through, offering thick, moving escape. The park, with bone-white trees snaking high against the crystal blue, the city laid out below as if a backdrop and not real. We lose ourselves in tracks that lead through the woods; take photos where we smile, the light wiping our features clean.

You take me to these places and I think of you alone here, thinking of me. We've made it to the other side of something challenging, seemingly insurmountable, and I smile inside, feeling I've won.

We dine with your new work colleagues – your brash boss, who talks too loud about his swimming pool, invites us on his boat. The women who work with you at your remote camp in the desert – the way they sit, leaning forwards on their knees with open legs, is mannish and unthreatening.

Your air-conditioned office, where all sorts of machines lie, waiting to be used for important work. I meet the receptionist you'd mentioned who'd seemed pretty and coquettish online, but is plain in real life. I feel foolish for worrying your head would turn.

We eat at a Chinese restaurant and I use chopsticks, feeling clumsy. Your boss shows me how to hold them, demonstrates picking up a single grain of rice.

'So what do you think of Perth?' he asks.

'It's great,' I say.

'He's getting on well,' he says, gesturing at you. 'But don't tell him that.'

You smile and so do I.

Your boss claps you on the back, raises a glass.

'To reunions,' he says, and winks. 'He's missed you.'

I feel foolish for being pleased, when he can't really know how you feel inside, late at night, alone.

You take time off and we drive down south, leaving the city behind. The sun fades, dancing in the high green leaves of ancient, wiry trees. We wind down the windows, stop for fish and chips along the coast. Bask in the balmy evening, sitting on the pier, looking out on shark-infested waters.

We're still hungry with the novelty of each other: always we have hands on knees, stroking inner thighs in the car, arms wrapped around each other on the sofa, spoon-like hugs as we break from cooking dinner.

We reach the town after dark and though I try to make it out, I can't. We drive to Tranquility Woodland, where you've booked a dated cottage. You're excited, pleased with this secret thing you've planned for me, and it's thrilling to be the object of a surprise. Carried away on the high of it, I have a sudden thought you might propose and wonder what I'd say. I'm horrified and thrilled – it feels too soon, but would still feel like a victory.

I'm always torn between wanting to reach a finish line, to secure you indefinitely, and at the exact same moment wanting the freedom of my own life, my own mind.

There is an outdoor bath and we drink champagne while it fills. We don't bother with bathing suits, and soon my hands are on your wet chest, searching under the water to where you are already hard. I look around the dark of foliage, the blackness of the sky, where watching eyes might wait, but I don't care. I smile at you, audacious with the power of being this person, and feel you harden more.

The next day we explore the wineries, find one we like and buy a case. The thought that I'm here long enough to drink it all with you is exciting. We eat a cheese board at a farm that makes it, sitting in their garden, watching a kookaburra in the trees. We visit the chocolate factory and eat too many free samples. Hide amongst kangaroo paws in the grounds.

That night, a bilby visits our patio and I get too excited and startle it away. Sleeping together is still a novelty and despite the heat we wake entwined.

I lie on the beach watching the waves crash.

You've gone back to work away – driving for days into the desert to a remote camp, exploring the surrounding area and mapping the land, looking for signs of minerals to exploit.

After London, the speed of life here jars, as if I have been running through air and have hit a wall of honey to be waded through. I pace the streets, feeling annoyed at slow-moving passers-by, then questioning why I'm in a rush at all. I have nowhere to go. I'm taking pause from some race I've been running all my life, and there's relief in it but also fear. I want a life so full it bursts at the seams; I have a dull sense that slowing down is not the way to achieve it.

I look for jobs although I have savings. I find one selling advertising in a construction magazine. I cold-call busy working men and manage to disarm them, keeping them on the phone until they succumb. I get them to do things they don't want to and I feel a buzz.

I'm wasting energy on this. I should be focusing on who I really want to be. I am torn between devoting time to that and showing you that I'm not some albatross you'll have to drag around; that I will support myself, if we decide I should stay here with you. It's what I want, but we don't talk about it – the fact that I am leaving in two months, attempting to enjoy each moment together. I don't ask you what you want and you don't ask me to stay.

I work on my novel, settling at my computer in the evenings and on days off. I'm too close to it and have to dig deep to know what to do. I overcomplicate it, then strip it back and worry I've removed too much.

Something within me – malevolent, dark – holds me to account. It's the antithesis of the surface person I've curated – carefree – and sometimes I wonder if it's the real me, hidden even from myself under some happy, smiling disguise.

It's lonely, but when I'm not at my computer, it's where I long to be.

This life feels like a dress rehearsal for something real that will come later – when I'm a writer. Even when I'm doing other things – cleaning the house, grocery shopping, cycling to work – my interior world is in a future where I stand on stage, hold my book, shake hands with readers.

Finally, I send the book to some literary agents in London and wait – terrified of silence or the wrong sort of noise. I wonder if my life will absorb into yours. Will my ambition dissipate in the sun or float away? I feel I must keep hold of it, like the string of a helium balloon.

As I sit on the white sandy beach, toes embedded in dust-like sand, I watch the families lay out picnic rugs and chairs, watch mothers swathe their kids in sun cream before themselves. The children run towards the sea in armbands, skin covered in swimsuits, hats. I wonder – could that be us? Could this really be our life? We're trying it on for size – cycling to the beach after work, submerging ourselves as the sun dips red-gold below the horizon as if it too is cooling off. The waves are big and we jump over them. I take a deep breath and follow you.

What is it that I want? I imagine myself, breathing in the smell of children's hair, bathing them and putting them to bed. Preparing packed lunches and all the clichés of a family life. Playing imaginary games with them, as I used to with my sister.

I see us too, standing tall and proud together, taking on the world. Boarding rickety boats to white-sand islands, being free. I see myself on stage, held up under lights. Can I have both, together, all at once?

We find our 'favourite' restaurant, a little tapas place in a row of trendy shops. The waiter is friendly, giving us sangria recommendations, and we drink too much.

'I'm glad you came out here,' you say.

'Me too. I can see why you like it.'

You move a garlic prawn around your plate. 'Do you? Like it?'

'Yes,' I say. 'I think I do.'

'Could you live here?'

Was that an invitation?

'I think so.'

'But what about London?'

'I could write from here. There's a small publishing house – perhaps they need an editor.'

You nod, avoiding my eye.

'Would you want me to?' I ask.

'Of course,' you say, looking up, taking my hand.

'You haven't asked,' I say. 'I wasn't sure.'

'I don't want to push you. It's up to you.'

'I need to know you want me here.'

'I do.'

'Are you sure?'

'Of course. I can't ask you to change your life.'

'I'd like to, I think.'

'Let's do it then.'

You reach over the table, kiss me. I feel a flood of relief, my limbo over – the decision finally made.

Drive

2011

We return to England for Christmas, drizzle and frowning, surly passport officers signals of home. We hire a car and travel around the country, seeing friends and family, spending hours on the road, side by side.

We mock the grey skies and bad coffee at motorway services. We miss the sunshine. We have adapted, acclimatised, and are proud of this.

Those hours in the car, music playing, we feel our difference from the people we come home to visit. Their lives are still the same, while we have moved, struggled, made friends, found jobs, ten thousand miles away.

We feel our lives spread out ahead of us, like we have all the time in the world.

We talk. We have time together in our bubble, and we talk.

You ask me questions you asked years ago.

You ask me to tell you about my fantasies. You ask me about women.

I feel the scrutiny of your words. Though I am afraid of the answers, I breathe in, and I hear myself speak.

I tell you about her. I tell you everything.

You listen. You are turned on. I notice, but I stay in my story, hearing the words I have kept inside me dissipate into the stale air of the long journey.

'Would you want something to happen now?' you ask.

I shake my head. 'It's too late now,' I say. 'I've found you.'

'It seems a shame,' you say. 'To never know.'

I think about her. About kissing the French girl at university, half-joking. About all those frustrated feelings I've had, I've feared. What would it mean if they were real?

I look at you. What if I open one door, and must shut this one?

I know I want you. I know I'm attracted to you. I know that's not a lie.

It's still a terrifying thought, to risk the fabric of our lives.

'I don't want to,' I say, and though you know that's not true, you nod your head.

I go to London and stay with my friend.

We're together again, under a spinning mirrored ball, our feet tacky on the sticky floor. I take my heels off and dance until my soles are black.

I've missed you, we shout into each other's ears, smiles spread wide, lit with cascading lights.

We try to make things how they were when we were young and free. But it's like trying to press the wrong jigsaw piece into the last space on the board. There's something false: a gap has formed between us that I can't get purchase on. I try to explain our life away: the endless sunshine, the beach, but every word becomes a sunlit cliché. I worry that she thinks I'm boasting, so I tell her the hard bits too: the lonely walks when you're away, the terrible waiting for something to happen with the book, the job that consumes my mind and my time. Staring up at white-limbed trees against a crystal-blue sky, having everything and nothing all at once.

She talks of London: of the shared flat she's moved to where she doesn't know the people well, the walls studded with photos of us. She looks tired, her skin tinged grey, her makeup more visible than usual. She takes me to the latest dim sum restaurant, and I eat too many glutinous balls to show her how great I think her life is.

She's single now. There's always someone she's waiting for a text from, some man who won't quite be who she wants him to be. We talk tactics, but I can tell she thinks I don't understand. I wonder if she thinks I'm smug, like those awful couples we used to mock, who become one inadequate person, clinging to each other like some ghastly four-legged creature. I complain about you just to try to show I'm not like that, and then feel bad.

'How's work?' I ask.

She shrugs. 'Good, I suppose.'

She never tells me much about her job – I'm not sure if it's become too complex to explain or if she just doesn't want to talk about it.

'Are you dating?'

'Yes.'

'Have you seen your ex?'

'No,' she says. 'It wasn't good, at the end. I found out he cheated on me at a party, but by then I'd cheated on him anyway.' She pauses. 'There's a guy at work.'

'Really?' I ask, imagining the boss – someone with power and danger attached.

'He's younger,' she says. 'It's a bit of a power trip.'

'Sounds fun.'

'It is.'

We meet her other friend – single, dressed in clingy revealing clothes, her lips painted red and smiling wide as she kisses me on both cheeks. *I've heard so much about you.* I watch them at the bar, laughing with heads bent towards each other. *That could be me*, I think. If I chose this life, I could still be with her, taking on the world. This city is now theirs, and I am an intruder, a passing visitor.

I dance alongside them, but something marks me apart and I feel alone.

You and I go to meet your best university friend, hugging him in a bar near his office, in a sleek, rich part of town. You mock his expensive suit and white shirt, asking where his trackie bottoms are. It feels very grown-up to have such serious friends.

The pub is crowded with people like us. It's Christmastime and the whole place glows. People enter stamping feet and exuding steam from warm mouths eager for a drink, shouting across the din to old friends. Someone has hung holly on the lintel above a roaring fire. I notice the ancientness of things: the old worn stone beneath my feet, the wooden beams above my head. The small English details that have gone unnoticed all my life are bright with difference now.

We drink pints and chat and laugh. This is your friend with whom you are your most playful self: less serious through being known so well. We express ourselves through sarcasm and wit, something I've missed. Communication is easier here and I wonder if that's what home is.

He's invited a colleague to join us: a blonde Australian girl who kisses us on both cheeks before queuing at the bar. I watch her tight-skirted arse and see her smile at the bartender. She is far from home as well, making her way in this big bright city, and this draws me close to her. When she returns, we talk of the excitement of being away from those we know, the thrill of building lives with no judgement or restraints. We smile and I feel lightning skip between us. As she speaks, I find my eyes watching her mouth, wondering what her lips would feel like on mine.

'What are you guys doing next?' she asks.

We all shrug — unencumbered, free, with no idea this stage of life won't last forever. This was supposed to be a quiet drink before dinner but it's almost nine already. I'm high on alcohol and an empty stomach. We order more drinks and bags of crisps, splitting them open to share, inhaling them, then ordering more. She and I steal outside for a cigarette, wrapping ourselves in coats and scarves, drawing close against the cold. She cadges a couple from some men-in-suits: so generic they make me laugh. I try to explain, and she laughs too, at the rolling conveyor belt of life around us. She lights my cigarette with the end of hers, leaning in. I see each eyelash brush her cheek and want to reach over and run my finger down her jaw. There is a silence as we hold eye contact, heavy with something I remember from long ago.

'Let's go out,' she says, exhaling smoke.

We drag the boys to a club she knows, but they are busy reminiscing, nursing pints. We shrug and say we'll meet them there. We walk fast through streets dripping with Christmas lights, giant toys and candy canes hanging above our heads. There's an urgency, as if we're afraid to lose this connection we've found which seems important, fragile. At the door of the club, she's waved past the queue, kissing the bouncer on both cheeks, and I wonder whether she's always so wild and free.

Inside, we find a booth. The boys join, complaining

about the entry fee, impressed that we didn't pay. We leave them to go and dance. Hidden in the throng of moving bodies, we look at each other: before I know it, we start to kiss. Her mouth is small and soft; her hands around my neck are light and gentle. There's something absorbing about her difference, and though I know I should stop, I can't.

'Let's go home,' she whispers in my ear, and I think – what is happening here?

You and I go back to the booth and she and your friend go to the bar for drinks.

'She just kissed me,' I say to you, and your surprise doubles mine. I feel bad about giving her the blame, but I'm unsure how you'll react.

'I think she wants to come home with us,' I say. 'What do you think?'

We leave your friend to take a taxi home. We're laughing, holding hands. When we get back to the apartment we've rented, I don't know what to do. Things feel different in the small, soulless kitchen. We have a drink and then she says she might go to bed. We offer her the sofa and, sadly, move into our room.

Under the covers, in the darkness, you reach for me. Turned on, you say, 'Do you think she wanted us?'

She wanted me, I think, but do not say. 'Yes,' I say instead.

'Go and get her,' you say.

I feel my stomach drop, unsure I am bold enough

to walk in there and do this. But I fizz with built-up want, and so I pull the duvet back and pad across the wooden floor towards her sleeping in the dark. It feels transgressive to sit down beside her, unsure if she's awake. I find her hand and feel her squeeze, pulling herself up and kissing me. Without the eyes around us in the club, we lose ourselves in each other. First, just our mouths and kissing is enough, but hands begin to wander and I find mine moving into her underwear. She tilts her hips, inviting my fingers in, and the wetness there is soft and yielding.

I hear the door creak open – looking up, you're standing outlined in dim light in boxer shorts. The questioning, eager look on your face makes my insides turn. We break apart, as if we were doing something wrong. You turn and walk away.

'I think he wanted to join in,' I say, expecting her to nod, to agree.

Her eyes are wide. 'I feel bad for him.'

I don't know what to say. I wonder why she's here if it's not for both of us.

'I think I'm going to go,' she says, kissing me on the cheek, gathering her things.

I see her to the door; we hug and then she's gone.

You are under the covers when I return to the bedroom, pretending to be asleep. I slide in beside you, unsure what to say.

'She's gone,' I murmur, into the deep silence.

'I was waiting for you for ages,' you say, eventually.

It didn't feel that long, but perhaps it was.

'I'm sorry. I was waiting for the right moment to come and get you.'

'I'm not sure that's true. You looked like you'd forgotten all about me.'

I remember being caught by something unstoppable, unavoidable, like white water rapids. I was a boat, tossed on the surface. Stopping felt futile, impossible.

'It felt strange,' you say. 'To see you with someone else. I didn't like it.'

I feel your anger radiating, your sadness. I've never seen you like this. I suppose I've always done things right.

'I'm sorry,' I say again, but you don't answer. After a while, I stop expecting you to, left only with the deep darkness of the bedroom, and the panic of having gone too far. Eyes open, I wonder if I've ruined things. My body thrums with fear and the shadow of my unfulfilled desire.

In the morning, I draw you towards me, determined to find my way back to you. I kiss you, and you resist then let me in. I hold your hands by your sides and rub my body against yours, my breasts edging along your chest. I take you in my hand and hold you there, feeling you harden.

'I love you,' I say. 'I'm sorry.'

*

Later, in the kitchen, we make coffee, and sit by the window looking over the city.

'I really was going to come and get you,' I say. I was, I'm sure I was.

You nod. 'I know. It's not how I imagined it.'

'Me neither,' I say.

'I suppose it's called a fantasy for a reason.'

I smile. 'We can tick it off our bucket list, at least.'

We sip, looking out. I think of how I felt last night. It was forbidden, but it felt right. I want to tell you how much I wanted her, to talk it through with you. This monumental shift – what does it mean? I think I do like women, but what does that mean for us?

I watch you, the curve of your brow, the tightness in your jaw, and feel a rush of love for who you are. I want you too.

You are more important to me than anything else.

Picket Fence

2012

The house we find is in a wisp of suburban Perth, a jacaranda-lined road full of wooden clapboard houses, white picket fences and scorched front lawns. We take photos of me hugging the street sign, pointing at the driveway leading to a complex of four identical grey houses with pitched roofs and porches.

It's mainly furnished, but we go to IKEA to buy a bookshelf for my office. We argue about which shade and despite my insistence, you turn out to be right. We make friends over Swedish hot dogs and you appease me by allowing the purchase of more kitchen utensils than we really need. In the heat, carting the items in and out of the car is strenuous and our tempers fray.

I watch your head bent over the flatpack instructions and wait for you to tell me what to do, but you don't, so I busy myself with unpacking other things. I'm learning that you like a plan, a structure, that efficiency is more important to you than feelings or fun. At first, I can't understand it: life seems too short for serious things.

We cook dinner in our tiny kitchen and start a routine that will last for years. I'm in charge of music, of tidying and laying the table, of washing up – the small menial tasks that surround the major one: the cooking. You never follow recipes, just throw things together, and I learn to trust your way with flavours, feel grateful for your skills, which mean we always eat delicious food.

'Where did you learn to cook?' I ask.

'My mum,' you say.

I imagine the chubby child I've seen in photos, the youngest one, bored at home while older siblings live their lives, following your mother around the kitchen.

'I'm glad you did,' I say.

When you return from camp, sometimes I get trussed up in lingerie and wait for you on the sofa. No matter how tired you are, how dirty from the desert, your eyes light up, you put your arms around me, lift me up, and carry me up to bed. I take my time, not rushing to get to the next thing – two weeks apart creates spaces I want to fill. I prepare, applying makeup, removing body hair, tidying the house, so I am ready for your return.

I am waiting, perfect, and you comply. You take control of me. We kiss, I wrap my legs around you. You drop me on the bed, and I am open, filled up with the thrill of being wanted, being enough. I am a participant but not the active one.

We whisper things to each other in the dark. You tell me about the girl behind the bar in the country inn you were staying in who knocked on your door, late at night, asking to come in. You tell me you turned her away, then touched yourself.

'Tell me you let her in,' I hear myself say. 'Tell me what you did to her.'

You talk slowly about touching her body. I feel the fear of it run through me as I imagine losing you to someone else, someone trivial. I grasp onto you, my prize, my special thing. I kiss you harder and we fuck inside the fantasy, safe in the knowledge that it's not real.

I contact the publishing house and am invited for an interview.

The office sits on the river's edge, overlooking the city in an old brick mill. Big arched windows frame the water and the glimmer of the skyline beyond. There are books everywhere – the coloured spines, the smell; it's glorious.

I get the job as an editorial assistant, catching the train each day. The tracks follow the river and then the sea and the view is light on water, sheltered by palms. I drink it in – the goldenness, the sounds of cockatoos in the trees. Each new strange thing brings me out of myself, reminds me life is wonderful.

Underneath, I am still waiting. I distract myself with other people's writing, honing their words and helping them prepare for publication. It's satisfying and takes my mind off the silence from the agencies. I hear from some – nice, lengthy rejections that are almost worse than nothing at all.

'How long will you continue to try?' friends ask, and I do not know the answer. I can't imagine giving up, but slowly, I fill my time with other things and the draw to the page begins to dull. We're busy making a life out in the sun, together.

We make friends – the South Africans who live across the lane, who make biltong in the garage. He's obsessed with barbeques and asks us round. We bring wine, and his wife and I sit in the sun while the men stoke and cook the food. I meet a group of women: we go to the cinema, beach – take trips away, and I start to feel I really live here. You play rugby – all your teammates seem like some male Australian caricature, throwing another shrimp on the barbie and downing beer. We hold a Halloween party and I make themed cocktails and canapés.

We frequent a local farmers' market, where the produce is cheap and fresh and we can buy meat in bulk. I take photos of dragon fruit – anything it's hard to find in England. We buy a scaly, hard-shelled durian and crack it open at home, bonding over how disgusting the strange yellow foetuses inside smell

We spend quality time together, visiting vineyards, walking into town to eat a piece of cake in the café with a hundred lampshades. We buy a bucket of chips and sit in the sun with beers, or eat pizza on the docks. Being so far away from home means we find home within each other and teaches me that wherever we are, we will be happy.

Trying

2013

We return to England, triumphant, for our wedding.

The castle-like hotel, the invitations sent, the Big White Dress. When we drive into the grounds of the hotel, I feel so lucky – untouchable – to have everything I've always wanted.

The night before, we risk bad luck: I sneak into your room on the other side of the hotel.

We open the bottle of champagne they've left in your room and drink it in mugs meant for tea or coffee.

We're gleeful, high on what we have together.

We find each other atop the sinking space of the hotel bed. Our bodies seem to fit. It feels like it did after we told each other we loved each other for the first time. We're reiterating and protecting what we have together, reminding ourselves of the strength of our bond, something only we can understand. I smile, wondering if this feeling flooding through my body is what creates new life.

The next morning, I wake early, returning to my room. There is a schedule to attend to. I watch my face transform in the mirror, wearing a dressing gown emblazoned with my new initials.

I left you in a haze of sleep and wonder what you're doing, thinking, feeling. I have a niggling fear that you will overthink things like you did once before, and I long to remind you who we are now, and who we will be, after.

I don't want to fall at the final hurdle, not understanding that this is a beginning, not an ending.

My mother helps me into my dress in the bathroom. The photographer captures the moment my best friend sees it, the bright wistfulness in her eyes. It's a photo I chose out of thousands to print and put up in our house – I'm not sure whether it's because it's full of joy, or evidence that I was one step ahead on the game of life.

I am the first and feel I've won some sort of race, that nothing in my life will stop my train, believing foolishly that I am behind the wheel.

I walk towards you in the church, and your eyes reflect my happiness back at me. Feeling my father's arm on mine, I take each step carefully, slowly, as I've been shown.

We really mean the vows we say in bright, cloudless voices. We look into each other's eyes, promising to love only one another. The words we speak feel solid now – immutable – prescribed in law.

They raise their glasses to our union, to becoming one, their faces joyful and resigned.

We'll be different, we say to each other.

We think that we have reached a finish line; our hands over each other's hold the knife, becoming one to cut the wedding cake.

Moving back to England feels inevitable, right: we've had our big adventure and now we'll be serious and settle down, starting a family close to home.

We move in with your parents at the farmhouse while we look for our own place. I spend the days walking in the fields, ironing whatever I find in the basket, helping your mother prepare dinner. We start drinking early, turning up the radio in the kitchen.

You help your father on the farm, busying yourself with tidying the dishevelled yard when he fails to give you jobs to do. You drive out together to check the sheep, off-roading the Land Rover easily onto grass, circulating the moving animals.

I see a house from a child's drawing – drawn square, with four windows and a coil of smoke escaping from a chimney. Roses around the door, in a quiet, field-swamped village. I imagine a stack of shoes beside the door, too many coats clustered together on pegs. On the fridge are children's scrawls, swimming certificates, school reports. A house of noise, of rosy moments, messy faces, braiding hair, Lego on the carpet – and not a moment's peace.

None of the houses we look at quite fit the brief – they all belong to solo couples whose children have left.

They rattle around in rooms too large, and seem sick of the sight of each other. I look at you and wonder if we'll end up there. I desperately want what everyone else has, and am simultaneously repelled by it.

After a few weeks, we find the one: a house of golden crumbling stone, like shortbread dipped in tea. A beautiful arched window lets light pour into the hall and down the stairs; the kitchen has an Aga and stone floors, the perfect place for baking bread and listening to Radio 4. A study with a fireplace where I can write, which I think secretly of forfeiting for a children's playroom.

As we walk around, I squeeze your hand. It fits the picture in my mind of what our life should be, a place we can have all the things we're told will make us happy, coveting the contentment of an ordinary life.

The first furniture-less night, we drink wine by the fire. You kiss me on the only rug we have and we make love, without protection, hoping for the best.

We move in gradually, unpacking boxes, stealing furniture from parents, friends. I unpack all my books, colour-coordinating the living-room shelves.

Your sister and I attend a course and I learn to use a sewing machine, playing at learning wifely skills. We get lost on the way there, careering down country lanes with music loud. I leave the sewing machine out in full view, evidence of this new person in this new life.

There is a distracting thrill in playing house together. I wear an apron and cook scones, serving them on a tray with a teapot and proper cups. When friends come to visit, I offer them home-baked bread. They mock me but I can tell they want my life. You fry bacon and eggs on the Aga top, cook tomatoes and serve a feast.

Those first few months, I'm eager, confident – *we're trying*, I say to people, not thinking failure possible. You warn me not to tell too many people, just in case, but I shrug you off.

As the months tick by, I berate myself for not trying hard enough. Sex becomes a game, something to be manipulated until the outcome suits. The lingerie is gone – I want you inside me for a different reason now.

When you find me crying in the kitchen, you kiss me on the head, tell me to let nature take its course.

I try, I really do. I take a job at a local magazine, writing lifestyle pieces about local furniture makers and the best pub walks. In my lunch break, I avoid googling phantom pregnancy symptoms – sore breasts, early pregnancy, when does nausea start. I attempt to stay away from forums of other desperate women – TTC, IVF – acronyms I don't want to know, don't want to be defined by.

Every time I get my period, I feel a failure and a fool. I hate myself for caring so much, but I do. You understand, but don't feel it as deeply as I do, don't want to talk about it as much. I see the resistance in your eyes and stop. There's nowhere else for these thoughts to go so I bury them deep inside.

I'm sure, at the beginning, that I will outsmart my body, that I'll be able to work my way around this, as I have with every other achievement in my life. I will win this race, as I've won all the others.

Your sister invites me to a Tupperware party at her house. We all bring a bottle and are subtly bullied into buying plastic tubs we do not need.

'You're the brother's wife?' a tall, willowy woman asks.

I nod.

'I've always had a crush on him,' she says.

I laugh, feel proud.

'It's nice to have a night off,' a round-bodied ginger woman says. 'Those kids are driving me mad.'

They all jump in, one after the other. I stay silent.

'How old are yours?' someone asks me.

'We don't have any yet,' I say.

'Yet,' another says. 'How old are you?'

'Twenty-seven,' I say.

'Plenty of time, then.'

Another woman clutches a pregnant stomach, complaining of sickness, of not being able to eat rare steaks. I want to shake her. Instead, I buy some plastic tubs and go home early.

*

I do all the things I didn't want to do: I take my temperature, I squat over my fingers to see if my cervix is open, I buy ovulation tests. I buy books and read them secretly, during the day when you're out at work, not wanting you to know the depth of my obsession. I want to be the easy, breezy person you married.

I print out an ovulation chart and hide it in a bottom drawer. I fill it in each day, and on the days when I should be releasing eggs, I pounce on you.

One morning, I walk across the fields and start to weep. The pain feels bottomless. I long for it to end, desperate not to be in this position. I'm mourning something that I've never had, and might yet have. That noisy house, full of mess, the clamouring hands, reaching for me. It's more than that: the first time I have failed and sheer will is not enough to put it right.

I try not to feel it so deeply.

I try to listen to you when you say we just need more time, to relax and let it happen, but my pain is sharp and deep, and will not be overlooked.

When your oldest friend comes round to announce his news, a bottle of champagne clutched in his hand, I smile to cover up my anger when I look at her, conspicuously not drinking.

I call my friend to talk about it, but it's impossible for her to understand. She tells me to be patient, that it will happen in time. I can hear her thinking – look at all the other things you have, but not saying that out loud.

I find solace in the women in chat rooms, who never tire of hearing the minutiae of symptoms, temperatures, sadness, but it is like an addiction to painkillers – numbing, but really exacerbating things.

I begin to know my body in different ways. I observe each small change: a twinge here, an imagined nausea there. I look for them, desperately. The heaviness of bleeding brings sadness, grief for something that happened only in my mind.

I long to feel my body adapt to new life. But it remains as it has always been: stubbornly repeating its monthly cycle.

My body becomes an adversary, a foe.

Something that must be appeased.

When you touch my skin, reaching out for me when we're on the sofa, in a neutral space, I feel myself recoil. I am steeling myself against pain, against you.

I can see you don't understand this, but I can't change it.

I don't want you anymore: I want what your body can offer me.

This must be hard for you, but protecting myself, doing everything necessary to have a baby, feels more important.

Later, I think. *I'll deal with your feelings later.*

We are prodded and poked. We sit in sterile beige rooms and wait with other depressed couples. We become a cliché, a story I have read about and turned away from a hundred times, thinking it wouldn't happen to me.

You hold my hand while my womb is filled with dye.

'I can't see a problem, but don't tell them I told you that,' a nurse winks over her mask, and I want to scream. I want there to be a problem, easily solved. A blockage, some simple reason this is not happening for us.

We rush a sperm sample into the hospital before the time window elapses. We get stuck in traffic and sit, tense, with the radio droning on. You get out of the car and run it in. When I pick you up, you're sweating, silent.

It's been hard to know how much you want this – looking at your tense, tight face, I see perhaps you do.

'I didn't want the results to be wrong,' you say.

We go for coffee and try to be the people we were before. We try to enjoy the city, to smile at the waitress and feel joy in small moments.

'Do you ever think there's a reason it's not happened?' you say. 'Like nature is trying to tell us something.'

Nature hadn't crossed my mind. If I'd imagined anything, it had been some sort of dark creature, determined not to give me what I want. Testing me.

'It's amazing what they can do now, to make it happen,' I say.

'But what if there's nothing wrong?' you say.

I can't think about that yet, so I don't answer.

'Or what if there is something wrong with one of us? Won't that be difficult too?'

Sometimes, I wish I could switch off your brain, stop you thinking all the things I haven't taken the time to weigh up – too busy moving forwards, in any direction. You slow me down, force me to see what's really there.

'Let's cross that bridge when we come to it,' I say.

On the way home, I think about what you've said. What if there's something fundamentally wrong with me? I try to imagine it, examining myself to identify feelings. I would deal with it, I think.

What if it's you? I feel the weight of responsibility, to reassure you that I don't mind, that I love you no matter what.

Suddenly, I'm not so sure I want to know everything after all.

Off the Path

2015

We become tired of waiting and busy ourselves with other things. We remove the carpet and sand the original floor in the living room, painting it a virulent shade of green. We tackle the ancient window frames, repainting the wood, filling in spaces where they've begun to rot.

We take on room by room. I start sanding down and painting old pine furniture. We weed the garden, prune the roses. You mow the tiny patch of lawn, regravel the driveway with a neighbour.

We don't talk about it but the efforts feel overwrought – as if we're preparing for a baby – a family – that might never come. What else could we be getting ready for?

I try to remember before. I try to remember lying on the beach in the sun in Australia, running into the waves. I try to remember feeling free, kissing you as we walk back from our favourite restaurant in the warm air, you undoing the strap of my dress at my neck.

How I felt at the altar, looking into your eyes.

So sure of myself, of the future.

I try to be untouchable again, but inside, I feel fragile. I look for my foundations, but it's as if they've disappeared.

I worry that I will never be the same again.

I worry that what has happened has dulled my bright view of the world.

I worry that from here there will only be darkness and shades of grey.

Our friends come to visit with their children. They are on their way to a camping trip, the car rammed full of the detritus that comes with small kids.

The weather forecast is bad. He brushes it off, smiling.

'It will be good for the kids to struggle,' he says.

'Not good for us, though,' she says, and I watch them exchange glances.

I try to imagine us with two small children, packing up the car. I wonder how we would have come together and how we would have conflicted.

As their children fill our house with mess, smearing pureed food, spreading out their toys, I feel my chest constrict. Is this really what I want?

I hear of sleepless nights, of troubles feeding, and I start to see that the experience I've had on a pedestal — of being a mother — is like any other, full of light and shade.

I've only ever thought of my life with children; not in a desperate, rose-tinted, maternal way, but simply because it is what is expected. When I really think about what it means to have a child – the next twenty years given over to that project – my desire begins to wane.

We talk, over and over, about our options.

Should we push harder, or should we wait?

I research, research, research, looking for the answer in books and online.

But this is not a problem with a definitive, easy answer.

My body is still a place I don't feel safe.

When we go to bed, I don't want to have sex with you.

Lying there with you inside me, I look up at the ceiling and feel nothing. I move, make noises, pretend. Are we creating something? If not, why are we doing this?

I wonder where that safe space has gone between us, why I can't access it anymore.

I don't talk to you about this. I'm not sure how to explain.

You seem the same: you reach after me, you want me, you get hard for me. This makes me feel worse, makes the gap between us widen. And there is a gap. I don't want to point it out in case by some miracle you haven't noticed it.

When we have left limbo, when a decision has been landed on, I will try to find my way back.

Gradually, over time, things start to shift. It's as if I'm floating gradually away from the pain, existing outside it instead of within. Each month, it becomes easier to cope with. One month, my period comes without me anticipating it, and it feels like progress, like climbing up a hill and looking back to see the view.

The more time goes by, the more space is created. I walk in the fields each day, watching small nameless birds dart between the hedgerows. I light the fire and sit at my desk to write. We've moved to this place to have the perfect family life, and without that, I'm not sure it will be enough.

I begin to soften towards you. This is an effortful process. I long for a release of tension, for the feelings that have gone cold and hard to melt fast and overwhelm me. I long to feel things in my body again, other than sadness.

When we are readying for bed, I look at myself in the mirror and tell myself I have nothing to be afraid of. I try not to hold my breath as I enter the bedroom and see you, standing in front of the mirror. I can look at your body, and I can see it is beautiful. I can see it is mine. I know it has given me pleasure and a place to escape myself. I tell myself it can do that again.

I stand behind you and we are reflected in the long

mirror, together. I put my hands around your back and touch your chest, your torso. I feel your body respond to the touch, craving it, as if you have been out of the sun too long. I'm grateful that you haven't given up on us, but also overwhelmingly sad that I have withheld something that you need. Your body is the way you show you love me, and I have been unable to let you do that. It isn't my fault, or yours: it is just the way things have been. I'm sad for lost time as I reach for you, kissing your neck, trying to convey with my hands how much I've missed you. You turn around and kiss me, and we fall backwards onto the bed.

I try to be inside myself, inside this moment with you. But I am still floating above us, watching us from the outside. I hope you believe I am the same as I was before. I worry that I never will be, that I will have to live with this feeling of disconnection forever.

We pant and breathe and move together and I feel you come inside me. I feel relief flooding through me, and it's so similar to a rush of desire that I almost mistake it for the same thing.

Your father is frustrating you. By coming back here to work alongside him, you were offering him the opportunity to be the father he failed to be when you were a child. At every turn, he has been a disappointment. If you come to him with ideas for the future, he clams up. This silence is not something we're willing to bank our future on.

You are becoming tense as a result of pent-up emotions unexpressed. One night, after a stony dinner, I crack.

'What's wrong?' I say, though I think I know the answer.

'Nothing, I'm fine.'

'You've barely said a word all night.'

'I'm tired. I've been working all day.'

I move my wine glass on the table. 'Are you happy?' I ask.

You look at me, as if that's not an important question.

'Are you?' I repeat. 'Because life's too short for this.' I gesture between us, meaning the tension, the silence.

'I tried to speak to my father again today,' you say. 'About what we could do with the farm. He listened, and then he said he'd think about it, but I know he won't.'

'We need to make a different plan,' I say.

'What can we do? This is the life we've chosen.'

'We can do *something*,' I say. 'What do you want?'

'I don't know,' you say. 'But not this. Not forever.'

'Me neither.'

We fetch a pad of paper and start to make a list. We could move abroad again: South America, Asia, Africa. I imagine the sun on my face, being in a no-man's-land away from people we know. But you're not sure you want to go back to your old job, long weeks away in challenging terrain, working for a big company where you have little control.

Working on your dad's farm appealed because of the opportunity to make your mark. If your father isn't ready for that, perhaps we can find our own way.

'Where would we get the money?' you ask.

I gesture around the kitchen. 'We could sell this place,' I say. 'We'd have a deposit.'

'But this is your dream house.'

'It was,' I say. 'But if we're not going to have kids . . .'

'Are we? Not going to have kids?'

I'm not sure how to explain. 'I don't want to wait around for something to happen to me. To us. Especially if being here isn't making you happy. We should just do something else, and if I get pregnant, we'll make it work.'

You look at me, nod. 'Let's start looking then.'

We spend the evenings with our laptops on our knees.

We go to look at a fishery business, but when we arrive it's secluded, down a long track and little more than a garden shed.

One night, you find a small collection of holiday cottages on the edge of Scotland. The photos show what was a farmyard, with a farmhouse and a series of converted buildings where guests stay. There's some land with it, a small vegetable garden. It's in a beautiful valley, with crumbling drystone walls and a nearby village within walking distance.

'We should go and look at it,' I say.

So we do. We drive north, and I feel us on the road again already, escaping the tedium of standing still. It reminds me of trips we'd take from university, setting off and feeling as if we could go anywhere together.

We find our way to the yard, where an old sign hangs slightly off-kilter. It could do with a clean, with a fresh lick of paint. The yard is potholed and uneven.

The farmhouse is tired and in need of attention, but the holiday cottages are fairly newly renovated. There are beautiful views from every window. I imagine myself tidying them for new arrivals, greeting them in the courtyard.

We are given a tour of the empty barns. They are pale stone with long, arching beams.

You tap the walls, examine the roof, asking the right questions. I feel a rush of love for you, for your brain, grateful that your mind can think clearly.

Potential, the estate agent says. And I see you nod once, in agreement.

As we walk back towards the car, I imagine us here. I imagine our lives as busy and full, with no time to think, to worry about the other things we might want.

'What do you think?' I ask you on the way home.

'I liked it,' you say. 'Do we want to do it, though? That's the question.'

I look at your side profile. 'What else are we going to do?'

You smile. 'I suppose so.'

It's strange to be completely adrift, off plan. Without realising it, I've been following a path laid out before me my whole life. I am good at doing what is expected.

We are young, and we have our lives ahead of us.

What do we want them to look like?

There is a fear in floating away from the shore, from the other boats docked there. There is also an exhilaration. Anything could happen.

While you're at work on Monday, I call the banks. I decide to start at the top – imagining men like my father, sitting in glass-walled offices. I can charm them, and I do.

I hear myself giving coherence to our passion and I get a buzz from it. I hear my voice, determined and clear, feel some old part of me rise up.

If I can't do that, I think, *I can do this.*

She's met someone.

She's secretive about it at first, as she is about all good things, as if she's learnt to be cautious, not to trust things. It pains me that she's been hurt so many times, and I really hope that this one is different.

He moves into her tiny flat in Wimbledon, and we go and stay the night.

He bear-hugs me at the door. 'I've heard so much about you,' he says.

His face is lit up with friendliness and genuine warmth, and I like him immediately.

He cooks dinner in her small kitchen, and as we chat in the living room, we can hear him, cursing good-naturedly to himself.

'Are you all right, my love?' she says.

'Fine, fine,' he says.

'Shall I come and help?'

'No, won't be long.'

We smile at each other, and you sip your wine.

We sit on the floor to eat. He brings out steaming platters of Moroccan food, covers the coffee table in them. Mounds of parsley-crowned rice, okra with pomegranate seeds, a huge tagine of lamb stew.

'Wow, a feast,' I say. 'Thank you so much.'

'He's such a brilliant cook,' she says, and I watch her look at him and glow.

He asks questions about your dad's farm, genuine interest lighting up his face.

'We're thinking of moving,' I say, and she squeezes my arm.

'You didn't tell me that! Where to?'

'We've found a business in Scotland,' I say.

You describe it: the farmhouse we feel we could modernise, the income that is just enough to cover a loan, the potential in the disused buildings, the farmyard. I hear you talk about it and it suddenly feels real, like we might really rip up our perfectly stable lives and do something different. I feel an aching to be that person, who takes a risk and sees it all pay off.

'It sounds amazing,' he says, looking straight at her. 'Perhaps we could do something like that, one day.'

I see her glow and feel it ignite something in me: that strange happiness that comes from others' joy.

'What do you think?' she asks me when he clears the plates.

'He's great,' I say, and it's so wonderful to really mean it.

They marry in the summer at her family home near the beach.

It's a beautiful day, and she's as relaxed as she can be with her sister and her mother fussing around her. They get married outside in the garden – a perfect front lawn and the flower beds a work of art. Purples, pinks, blues and yellows: the colours glow under the rare English sunshine, and the grass is green and lush beneath our feet.

I do a reading – something she has chosen about love being more than surface, about building a life together – and as I read the words, I look at her, so radiant and happy. He is smiling through his beard. He has the sort of face that displays his every emotion, and right now I can read excitement, concern for her, and a little fear.

They buy a house outside London with an orchard

in a lovely village, and busy themselves with decorating, knocking down walls and adding rooms, putting their mark on the place. They waste not a single apple that first year, taking on the responsibility of collecting fallen ones each day as if their lives depend on it. I recognise her joy in simple things and feel it alongside.

She has been trying for a baby too and it hasn't been going well.

She's in that awful, dark hole. She calls me when her period comes, her voice breaks, and she is sobbing.

'I just feel so stupid,' she says.

'I know, I know,' I say.

I'm beyond that painful threshold now, but I remember and know the right things to say. Through shared pain, we find each other again, a closeness we haven't had since you and I first met. I'm grateful in a way, for these dark things that have brought us together.

She tries to call me one night, but I don't answer.

I call her back in the morning and she sounds strange, tense.

'I have to tell you something,' she says.

I know what it is before she says it.

'I'm pregnant.'

I wait for it: the rush of pain, the claustrophobia of finding the right reaction, but it doesn't arrive.

'That's great,' I say.

'Are you okay? I've been so worried about telling you.'

'I'm fine. Honestly. I'm happy for you.'

'Are you sure? I wouldn't be, if it was you.'

'I am, and if I'm honest, I'm so relieved. It would be so hard not to be able to be happy for you.'

I hear her exhale.

'How do you feel?' I ask.

'I'm happy, of course,' she says. 'But I'm almost afraid to be. What if it goes wrong? What if I let myself believe it, and it ends?'

'You can't think like that,' I say, though I understand.

'I know,' she says. 'I'm trying.'

When I get off the phone, I make myself sit for a moment, examine myself as if checking for injury, damage. I try to work out how I really feel, whether I'm masking jealousy, sadness, pain. But there's nothing there, or not that I can find.

New

2017

We move to the new house a few days after the New Year. It snows over Christmas, and it feels like the white world outside the window is readying for a new start too.

That night, I can't sleep, going over all the things I need to do tomorrow for the guests who are arriving, all the things I mustn't forget. We have put everything on the line to buy the place, and we can't afford to put a step wrong. After what feels like hours, I hear you sigh.

'Are you awake?' I ask.

'Yes.'

'What are you thinking about?'

'Just wondering if we've made a terrible mistake.'

'So was I,' I say, and we laugh.

You reach out for me, and somehow, being warm and close, skin touching, I feel better.

'We can do this,' I say.

'We're going to have to,' you reply.

The first guests have no idea that I have never done this before. I welcome them into the cottage and show them around: the different rooms, the settings for the heating and the oven. They ask me for a recommendation for a pub for dinner and I mention the one with the best reviews in the village, though I haven't yet had time to visit myself.

I drive out to the wholesaler to stock up on all the small necessities. It's in a huge warehouse on the outskirts of the city. It's cold and despite my coat, I feel exposed as I walk into the vast space. I learn to use the strange, bulky trolleys, filling them with boxes of mini jars of preserves, of huge stacks of toilet roll, of cleaning products.

I become used to coming here. I learn, embarrassingly slowly and in front of an audience of men, how to use a pallet lifter, how to drag it around the space without bumping into things. I learn how to find a porter to use his forklift to pick up my pallet and put it in the back of the van. I learn how to drive the van carefully, so the contents don't fly around in the back.

Readying the cottages is methodical and physical. I feel my body from dusting the highest shelves, from scrubbing the shower cubicle. I begin to enjoy the smell of bleach, the smoothing of things until they are neat and ready again. There is a pleasure in making everything look beautiful.

The days go by and we seem not to be sinking. When we have no guests I get used to the cloying feeling that we are doing something wrong, and learn to focus on the future, keeping myself busy with what this place could be. I make small improvements, collecting local produce from the butchers and bakers in the village, making up welcome hampers and packs of information for visitors. I paint the sign at the entrance.

Together, we scheme what we will do next. Over wine in the evening, we draw on old plans: turning old buildings into new cottages in our minds. We talk about renovating a larger barn for weddings. Finally, we have a place that is truly ours and we can make it whatever we like. There is a deliciousness about this ultimate freedom.

We clear the small vegetable plot on the first bright morning of the year. We turn the earth and dig up the weeds, readying it for new life. I lose moments working in silence beside you, my mind clear for what feels like the first time. The sun on our faces, the light glimmering from the new green on the trees, I look across at you and I feel happy.

We have our morning coffee together each day, sitting in the sunshine.

On rare quiet days, we walk up the fell behind the cottages, clambering over rocks and feeling heather rough beneath our hands. I breathe in the smell of damp wood and moss, the peculiar freshness of the air here. I feel sweat prickle as we climb higher; it is not such a steep slope, but I am wearing layers. When we reach the top, we look down and see the cottages from above, the farmyard, garden and barns seeming so much smaller from here, so much more manageable than when I am within them, working hard.

We sit in the evenings and drink deserved beer, chatting about our days. We try to celebrate small wins regularly, not knowing how long they'll last.

Our friends pop in on their way to places. We book out the cottages for them and enjoy long, leisurely meals we cook from scratch. They tell us they are proud of us for taking the leap, for doing something different.

We get to know the guests, some of whom return several times a year. It is a place they come to escape their lives: to sit on their small terraces and listen to the birds. They walk in the fields and give themselves permission to stop.

I see worry etched on people's faces as they check in. I am friendly, warm, and I find I am good at drawing them out, at making them feel comfortable. They tell me things they wouldn't tell a stranger. It makes me pause and consider the small trivialities that take up so much of my own energy. I feel a sense of relief wash over me, at this shared burden.

It also makes something solidify inside me — something I've always felt becoming crystallised. I don't want an ordinary life. I don't want to live inside the lines.

We walk through the small town we've moved to. Past the butchers, bakers, hardware store, fish and chip shop, pub.

Each day, we leave the intensity of the business and head towards the river: to the rushing water flowing through the town.

We stand side by side on an ancient stone bridge and look down into the water.

People begin to know our names. We are the new owners of the holiday cottages. We are no longer anonymous. Sometimes I feel as if I'm living inside a glass box. I long to fracture it, to blur the line of sight.

The business fills all our time, our minds, our bodies.

There is a relief in this.

It is a get-out-of-jail-free card.

There is also a reprieve from the pressure of sex.

We are both tired, falling into bed without thinking about touching each other, or what comes after. I feel freed from something for a while at least. The scrutiny of your want, which makes more visible the lack of mine.

A routine begins to form. It's as if we've been handed a huge ball of yarn to detangle, and slowly we are separating the single thread. The bookings, the tasks, the days begin to organise themselves around a repetitive pattern.

We take our first day off and drive to the seaside, crossing the flat, heather-rough moors. The sky stretches over our small car, and I feel the world enlarge. All this was here, all that time. I take your hand where it rests on the gear stick and squeeze. We walk along the windy beach in silence. The roar of the waves, the blistering cold, make my mind still and flat, and I relish it. I can feel you soaking it in too.

You begin to reach for me again. I am hopeful I will feel differently in this new place. I am a new person, in our brand-new life. But when you touch me it's the same as before. My body reacts before my mind. I watch your face constrict and the guilt rushes in.

I begin to feel dread as we head up the stairs, or earlier when we're eating dinner or watching television. I don't think about whether I want to have sex, just that you do and so I should. It feels like another task I must complete and I feel trapped by it. Once it's happening, I enjoy it and can loosen myself enough to let you in. I pretend too, betraying you as I make noises I don't really feel, knowing that the most important thing to you is the truth. It feels like the only option.

It's easy to blame this feeling on how busy we are, on how much I am holding in my mind, responsibilities like washing pegged on a line. I don't feel sexual at all, ever. There is always something more 'important' to do. I don't see physical pleasure as a priority. I think about this a lot. I think about the early days when we first got together, the deep well of longing I found inside myself. I think of the other men I've been with, kissing them on the dance floor and wanting to melt, to disappear into them. Why can't I find that feeling again?

Sometimes I worry that there's something fundamentally wrong with me. I even wonder if perhaps I am a lesbian. I think about her, about those intense feelings I had when we were teenagers. Sometimes, I think about our failed threesome, how I let myself be carried away by it. Was that how things are supposed to feel?

I remind myself of the early passion with you, and I tell myself that my deepest darkest fears must be wrong.

You never pressure me. Every time I see your face as I turn from you, I feel I am chipping away at something essential. I know I am not giving you what you need, but I can't. I simply can't. I worry about it, but push the thoughts away. You are collateral to a problem that is mine. I know that something has changed inside me.

As I go about my day, checking the online bookings, greeting guests, I think about this space within me where longing used to be. I try to locate it, unlock it again. I'm sure that if I solve the puzzle, it will click open and all the feelings I am supposed to have will rush towards me and everything will be as it was.

I meet her halfway between our houses. She brings the baby, who looks up at me from her bassinet, appraising me with those sardonic grey blue eyes I remember from the disco when we were fifteen.

The pub we meet at is nothing special — a convenient, equidistant location — but I know it will be marked out by our meeting here. We haven't seen each other in months.

I hold the baby on my knee while we chat; observe the solidity of her, her sudden movements. I've feared this moment on the journey here: that it would start up an ugly longing in me that I wouldn't be able to quell. I am grateful not to feel that.

She talks of dirty nappies, of little sleep.

'I've just moaned at you for half an hour,' she says, taking a sip of her lime and soda.

'You haven't,' I say. 'We're catching up.'

'I hope it's okay,' she says. 'To talk about the baby.'

'Of course it is,' I say. 'It's like seeing into a different world.'

'One full of shit and sleep deprivation.'

'And love, and life.'

She gives me a look. 'You make it sound so . . . rose-tinted.'

'Things always are, from the outside.'

'How are things with you?'

'Busy,' I say. 'The business has been manic.' It's hard to put into words the intensity of it, its pull on me. 'I just don't get a moment to myself.'

She nods. 'I know what you mean,' she says. 'I feel like that about the baby.'

I nod. 'I don't have the mental space for anything else. Like sex.'

'That's the last thing on my mind,' she says.

I feel relief.

*

Once our lives begin to steady themselves, we feel, alongside each other, a sense of real achievement. The doubts we both held, individually, about whether we could do this, are proved wrong and begin to lift. Like fog in a valley, once they dissipate, we can truly see what lies around us.

Each month, I check the bank balance, pay the bills. It remains the same, creeps slightly upwards some months. This feels enough, for now. The thought of making this work drives us forwards, makes us continue to try.

We reach some milestones: first six months, first year. Once we are in a routine, we begin to make progress. Together, we clear one of the other buildings for renovation. You become obsessed with underfloor heating, with structural walls, spending hours watching videos on YouTube. Your Instagram feed is a series of tedious DIY videos.

People tell us – friends, family, customers – that they are impressed by what we've achieved. I feel this praise land on my skin, like snow, but it doesn't feel necessary for it to sink in. I look at you and know we have worked hard, that we have done this.

We sell our old boring silver car and buy a small, second-hand convertible. We only need two seats, and there is a pleasure in this. In making decisions that aren't based on What-Ifs, or What-Might-Bes, but on what we want, now.

*

I start masturbating.

I try not to think too much about it, to stop myself before I start. My mind says wait – just fill the washing machine, fold those clothes, reply to those emails – and then you can do this other thing. But I am firm, and make myself do it.

I have a bath after a long day, and I sit in the water, trying to still my rushing mind.

I touch my own body and I wonder if this is the first time, ever. I know it isn't – that there have been many other times in the past, but it feels brand new, like a discovery.

Sometimes, I am too eager. Like coming across a deer in the woods, I startle it away.

I find my breasts and nipples, coaxing them to life.

I let myself go.

Mostly, I let my mind be blank, but things arise – images, real and imagined – and I let them come.

I rerun the things I used to fantasise about when I was a teenager. I am a maid, working in a rich couple's house. They make me clean their bedroom while they watch, and then the husband pleasures me, touching me gently, teasing me, while the wife looks on.

'You must not come,' he says, and this makes me come every time.

There's another fantasy, where I run away from home, arriving in a big city after dark. I don't know anyone. There's a woman who asks me if I have somewhere to stay. She offers to take me home with her, but it turns out her house is a brothel, and she is a madam. I must sing for my supper.

I start to realise that all my fantasies involve someone else taking control of my sexuality. I wonder why I am ashamed to be active, to be sexual. I wonder if I've always been waiting for someone else to take me by the hand and make me live – first her, now you. I wonder what it is I want, and I long to find out.

When I ask myself, I don't know the answer. I feel I need to act, but I'm not sure what to do.

I start to realise that I've been filling my life with tasks to distract me from how I really think and feel.

In quiet moments under the rush of the shower, I make my legs shake, muffling sounds with water flow. I hold the shower head between my legs and feel my mind say no.

This voice is so loud, I can't hear whether or not it is my own.

Making myself come helps me in the moments when we're together. When we go to bed, I close my eyes and reach for you. I allow my body to open up.

I want to be near you more now, too. These things we are achieving bind us together.

It makes it easier to talk to you about how I felt before and not frame it as a rejection of you.

You listen without judgement as I talk about how I didn't feel connected to my body, how I still don't sometimes.

I tell you about my afternoon delights, and you ask – what do you think about?

I try to find the words. I tell you about my fantasies, feeling they are small and childish, that you will find them foolish. But you don't. You ask if I want to act them out, but the thought repulses me.

'I don't know what I want,' I say. 'But I want to find out.'

'What about women?' you say.

Many of my fantasises involve women. If I watch porn, which I do rarely, I always search for girl-on-girl. I'm never sure if this is because of the crassness of other porn, the men hairless and sneering, the women's mouths open wet Os. When I watch these films I think of Barbie and Ken, of plastic, sterile moments I can't identify with.

'I think about women too,' I say.

'We could try another threesome,' you say.

I look at you, wondering if you're serious.

I try to imagine it, but I can't. 'I'm not sure,' I say.

I can't remember discussing it again, but we do. Many times. We have the same conversation over and over before we act.

I want to fan the small, beginning tendrils of lust I have found.

I remember saying that perhaps we should see what happens, as if finding a threesome is like stumbling across edible mushrooms in the forest. I remember you saying that nothing will happen unless we seek it out.

We both want something new here. We have proved in our new lives that we can be challenged and we can grow together. You are also an adventurer. It's what we have in common. And this will be a new adventure, an extension of what we do in the rest of our life together.

'How would we do it?' I say one night over a glass of wine.

'I don't know,' you say. 'Google?'

I laugh. This seems ridiculous. 'Google can't solve every problem, can it?'

You shrug. 'There's no harm in trying.' You pull out your phone. 'How to find a threesome . . .' you say, while typing.

We laugh.

You fall silent while you scroll.

'What does it say?'

'There are apps. Shall I download one?'

'There's no harm in that.'

I imagine a path leading into a dark wood, us taking the first step.

'We have to write a profile,' you say. You pass me the phone. A box on the screen: About Us at the top.

We're a married couple in our thirties, looking for a third to fulfil a fantasy.

I show you.

You type, pass me the screen.

We both love adventure and live life to the full. She's an editor, he's a geologist. Drop us a message to find out more.

'That's good,' I say. 'Except we're business owners now.'

'Decoy,' you wink.

I laugh.

You set the account to Private, add a photo of us smiling on the beach, and we wait.

Watching television, over weeks and months, you field messages and photos and show them to me. I say no until you hold up a photo taken on a balcony: she's wearing a yellow dress, is smiling at the camera. She looks normal, pretty.

'Yes,' I say.

We arrange to meet in a shopping centre on a midweek day. Leading up to it, I'm shocked at our audacity. I try to imagine us, walking past rows of shops, calmly meeting a stranger for coffee before potentially taking off our clothes and having sex with her.

It's exciting to turn the thought over, like a delicious boiled sweet. I reach for you on the sofa, squeeze your arm while we're watching television.

It's fun to have a secret. We have something to talk about which isn't the business. We have speculative conversations about something new.

Can we kiss her?

Can we fuck her?

Some of these questions are impossible to answer until we are inside the moment, until our feelings arise. Talking about them in the bright light of our kitchen over a glass of wine is not the same.

How will we communicate doubts?

What if one of us doesn't like her?

What if one of us is uncomfortable?

I am more worried about these things than you: I have always had more difficulty saying what I really think for fear of upsetting somebody.

That night, we have sex, as if reminding ourselves of something. As if by drawing close, we are protecting what we have, readying it for what might come.

In the car on the way there, my mind is full of doubts. Worst-case scenarios.

It feels like we're hurtling towards something that could destroy us.

This could be a funny story we tell at dinner parties, or it could be something cataclysmic.

In some ways, what happens in that room is everything I imagined. I had longed to want another woman again and I had feared it. I find the resolution to a question that has surrounded me like smoke for all my life. There is a huge relief in that.

The bigger relief comes from the grey areas I discover in those white sheets.

I want her, but I still want you. It is possible to want both at the same time. I start to wonder if this isn't about wanting men or wanting women at all. This is about wanting, in general.

My senses are heightened watching you with her: I feel the risk of it, but there is a joy in sharing what we have, in seeing you from the outside again. I watch you fuck her and I see you as a desirable person, someone I have ceased to see in our everyday lives. There is also a joy in being the architect of your pleasure, in being in control of it.

Afterwards, I feel a strange sense of euphoria. We walk back to the car, around ordinary things, and I am astounded that the world still turns the same.

We discuss it on the way home. The way we each felt. I try to describe my relief. You tell me how strange it was, to be with someone else after all this time, in front of me. But the words can't add up to the experience. We were there together. Our experiences were the same, but also utterly different.

Our individual versions of the truth are not what's important. What's important is that we felt aligned. We were completely in our experiences, but also connected to each other. I felt close to you when you were inside her, linked by your focus on me, as the real subject of your attention. I also felt freed by the fact that I am no longer the sole keeper of your pleasure.

I wonder if this feeling of connection is a fallacy,

but it feels real. It goes against everything I am told I should feel in this situation – shattered, broken, alone.

We both agree we want more. We want to try new things, in new places.

When we go to bed that night, you stand in front of the mirror. I see you with her, in my mind's eye, and I feel my heart speed up. I want you again because I saw her want you.

As we fall back together onto our bed, I feel as if she has handed me a gift.

PART II
Awakenings

White Party

2019

The taxi ducks through dark streets, tracing the path to an industrial estate out of town. I feel unmoored, as if the ropes that keep us in place are slipping, stretching, falling away.

Lights catch smears of red on the brick frontage as we pull up, splotches of colour in a black-and-white photograph. There is an open doorway, golden light, the outline of a man, standing tall, hands on hips. I squeeze your hand as you pay the taxi, and we look at each other, pulling our masks down onto our faces.

We step outside. It's the middle of summer, the air still sharp on my bare legs. There is the smell of smoke, though I'm not sure whether I imagine it as some overhang from an industrial age. The building looks like an old cotton mill, and I think of school history lessons, of children paid to risk hands pulling thread from machines.

'Are you ready?' you say, and I nod.

I imagine us, silhouetted, edges sharp in the soft light. Cardboard cutouts of a man and a woman in black tie, holding hands.

We have talked about this moment. I have pictured it, how it would feel, to be this person, inside a glamorous secret. It feels exciting, but also the precipice of something. We have been accepted, but I don't yet know if we are acceptable.

At the entrance, our IDs are checked, tickets shown. I hold my breath, imagining turning back. Instead, we're waved inside, where pretty girls in lingerie explain the rules – no phones, or photographs; masks on until 11pm.

We walk up a staircase, lit with candles. In the main room, a chandelier burns above our heads; a long red curtain blocks our view of half the room. Music plays: adult, sultry. A long, dark bar; small groups of people hover chatting. The shine of black patent heels against stone floors, the white-clad bodies strangely incongruent with the dark spaces.

We go to the bar and order G&Ts, make eye contact with another couple waiting, smile.

You introduce yourself – I'm impressed. They lean forwards, kiss us on the cheek.

She is wearing a tight-fitting white dress, has curling dark hair. He's shorter than her, with a broad smile. He steps from foot to foot, as if he has too much energy and it must escape.

Behind my mask, I long to see their faces, to show them mine.

'I like wearing the masks,' she says. 'It's seductive.'

'Me too,' I say, though I don't. I am finding I don't like to be told what to do.

'Is this your first time?'

'Yes,' I say. 'You?'

She smiles, teeth flashing. 'No, we've been before.'

I smile back and between our eyes I feel something fizz, and pop.

I look over at you. You're laughing with the other man. You've pulled your mask up on your forehead, and I can see your eyes, crinkled.

Behind you, people talk, holding drinks aloft. The big red curtain hiding something beyond it. Right now, it could be any bar, or party, anywhere.

Sometime later, she takes my hand and leads me to the toilets.

We go into a stall and she closes the door, pressing her back against it. I wonder for a moment if she might kiss me.

From our handbags, we pull out lingerie. There had been discussion of such practicalities in the chat group so I'm prepared. *Bring underwear, to change. BYO sex toys.* I unzip my white dress. I see her abs, her muscular legs, and wonder if my body is enough.

We help each other, attaching delicate belts to the thick lacy tops of the suspenders across our thighs. I feel her light fingers on my skin and swallow. She's taken off her mask and looks up at me with large amber eyes: my stomach dips and I know I want her.

In the mirror, we join a line of women, altered. We compliment, reapplying makeup, sharing lip gloss. I feel the familiar warmth of female spaces. I think of a marble bathroom, of the smell of sweet perfume.

I take her hand, feeling bold; she kisses my cheek.

We step out into the changed space of the club, finding the men where we left them by the bar. Still fully dressed, their eyes move up and down. I feel your eyebrows rise; you reach for me, and I feel your pride like a medal. We kiss like we used to, hungrily, before we belonged to each other, knowing they are watching. I still have her hand and pull her towards us, away from him. I kiss her softer lips, drawing them towards us. I feel his hand on my arse, his fingers moving slowly, and warmth spreads.

'Shall we explore?' I hear you say, and we all follow, towards the red curtain and what's beyond.

A row of beds along three walls.

Bodies already move there, but it isn't crowded yet. Some couples play, touching, hips shifting in and out, like cogs inside a smooth machine. We stand for a moment, watch.

A metal cage, curved like a shell. I touch the cold bars, the open door, thinking of Venus rising from the waves.

It's empty, and I step inside, reaching above my head

to hold the bars, feeling my body arch and stretch. I feel the heat of their eyes on me, the power of leading the way. She follows me inside, pulling herself up in front of me, pressing her small breasts against mine, kissing me as the men watch.

I pull her into me, my arms around her narrow body. She's small and soft and matches me; something about this just feels right. I feel the slide towards oblivion begin and I close my eyes, sinking. I feel her hands moving down my body, her fingers lightly brushing my nipples through the gauzy material of my lingerie. I swallow, feeling the electricity of my nerves reacting to her touch. She is slow and takes her time; I both long for urgency, for what comes next, and want each moment to last forever. She moves my underwear: I feel her tongue flick between my legs and hear myself cry out, pleasure washing through my body. Everything around us blurs and focuses into this clear moment. I reach for her hand and she squeezes as if she feels it too, this place we've found.

I can feel the eyes of the men, and others, watching from behind the cage. They are shadows without substance, seem unimportant. I don't care who can see.

You follow us in, moving behind her and kissing me. We surround her body with ours. He is there too, behind me: I feel his torso against my back. I turn slightly, kiss him, and taste mint and something deep and cool, like the smell of eucalyptus trees. His tongue moves fast, and I follow, though it feels out of sync. I want to put my hand on his chest and slow him down, but don't.

I let him take control and feel myself slip slowly, further from my pleasure, towards what I think he wants me to do. I become more aware of my surroundings: the beat of the music playing, the people watching us. I have moved from being inside to being outside, and I watch myself move down his body, undoing the buttons of his shirt, teasing him, my mouth moving slowly towards my destination. When I get there and unzip, though, he is not ready, and I wonder if he is outside too. I wonder how to get us back inside this moment, but I don't know the answer.

I take him in my mouth and hope he will get hard. When I look up, his eyes are closed, and I want him to look at me, to see. I can't communicate this, so I continue. I want what I had with her, with him. When he still struggles to get hard, I try harder, double down. I sit on top of him; I touch myself. I do things I have seen in porn. Men are supposed to be ready, to be eager, to be switched on. The more I try, the more I feel I am to blame.

After a while, he pulls away, laying me on the bed beside her, and moving his mouth between my legs. She and I lie together, side by side, the men below us, and kiss. I close my eyes and try to feel his tongue, the pleasure spread and deepen. He is good, but something disconnects.

*

Other things happen.

We find a space on the big bed and have sex, just us, in front of the room. I am on top of you and I rock back and forth, feeling eyes on my breasts. I am comfortable taking the lead with you and it feels good to be here, together, watched.

Soon, others join us, and we touch and play. We may never do this again, and I want to try everything, to soak it all in. But I also want to be alone with you, to discuss, to just be us.

The taxi takes us to a big white bed, and sleep.

We are buzzing and not yet ready to close our eyes. We are also ravenously hungry. We order pizza: you collect it from the hotel foyer, bringing it into the room as if you have made it yourself.

We devour it, naked under the sheets.

'Was it what you expected?' you say.

I pause. 'No. I think it was better.'

'In what way?'

'The people, I suppose. They were normal. Good-looking.'

'Were you expecting monsters?'

'I was expecting darkness.'

'Did you come?' you ask.

'Yes,' I say. 'With the girl at the beginning, in the cage. Did you?'

'No,' you say. 'There was a lot going on.'

I remember the room of bodies; seeing the huge,

ongoing mass of people moving had felt rare and strange, like seeing one of the wonders of the world.

'I know what you mean,' I say. I want to ask you about the man in the cage who didn't get hard, but I know what I am really asking is if I am sexy, if I am enough.

'We should go again,' I say, wanting another opportunity to try.

'Let's,' you say, and kiss me. Your mouth is so familiar, your taste, your tongue. It makes me smile, breaking the kiss.

'What?' you say, smiling too.

'I love you,' I say. 'That's all.'

'I love you too,' you say.

Waking in the hotel room on smushed sheets, I worry I smell like someone else. But you draw me towards you, kiss me despite my morning breath, and you are hard.

We look into each other's eyes. We dig nails, cling. We touch each other as if we don't know each other's bodies. We fuck lazily, spooning in the bed, and it's sensual, slow. There is such a relief in being back in a place I recognise.

We drive home through grey streets, normality feeling like a suit that no longer fits.

I squeeze your hand as we pull into our drive, our house an old friend.

Inside, I unpack our suitcases, washing my underwear in the sink and hanging it on the clothes horse inside, though the sun is shining. I don't want our customers to see some private part of who we are, something taboo that is unaccepted. I want to be proud of us for being bold and living outside the lines, but I also want my privacy to explore this new adventure, alone. I put our masks back in the drawer in the spare room, and I push the suitcases back under the bed.

I feel as if I am in a trance. I see myself stacking the dishwasher, but I also see her, the person I was in that dark room. I am the person that did those things, but I am also not. I am also the person sitting here now, in our house, in the normal world.

Hot Tub

2019

The patio is cracked; grass grows where grout should be. The hot tub sits, the water rippling. The small patch of lawn is overlooked, surrounded by a wooden fence that is not quite high enough.

There's no one outside so we knock on the glass doors and let ourselves in. Inside is dim – a long living room, small kitchen. Two people are sitting on a sofa and look round as we enter. She's wearing a cropped black top and pencil skirt and high high heels. Groomed identical brows, long straight hair, lined lips.

He looks serious, strong, and I imagine him holding someone down, then wonder why I'm not imagining me. He seems on guard, as if waiting for something bad to happen.

'Are you the hosts?' I ask.

He laughs. 'No, we've just arrived.'

'They're finishing something off upstairs,' she says. 'Said to help ourselves to a drink.' She shakes a prosecco glass at me, points over to the kitchen counter, where a bottle sweats.

I go and fill a glass, ask you what you'd like.

'Is there any beer?'

I open the fridge, when the hostess comes down the stairs.

'It's in the other fridge,' she says. 'I'm sorry. We ran out of time.'

She leans in to kiss me on the cheek – black hair, oval eyes, long neck – she is like a Modigliani painting.

Her accent is foreign, hard to place.

She goes to the garage, brings back two beers and hands them to the boys.

'We haven't even turned the lights on.'

She flicks the switch and the small space is thrown into light.

I look around the room as the others make small talk. A collage of magnets on the fridge, and along every windowsill and surface, small cactuses and other plants.

'My babies,' she says, seeing me looking. 'This one,' she picks up the one I was looking at, the pot no bigger than a fifty-pence piece. 'It's rare.'

'Where do you get them all?' I say.

'Online, mostly. It's my only vice.' She laughs, throatily, looks me right in the eye.

We're outside when more people arrive, sitting on makeshift seats around a futon on the floor. The hostess sits on it, cross-legged, asking questions, telling jokes. It feels like we're watching a one-man show.

Her partner finally emerges from the house. He is

thin and pale, wearing a shirt and jeans. I can tell his body is muscular from the stiff, proud way he holds it. He invites cold admiration.

She's apologised for him already, telling us how he likes everything to be perfect, so when I meet him, he seems tainted, flawed. She was joking, overblowing, but I still imagine him in a padded room, wearing a straitjacket.

A man in a chequered shirt arrives, apologising for being late, blaming his red-haired wife, who rolls her eyes.

'You were the one agonising about what to wear,' she says.

'I wanted to look my best.'

He takes guardianship of the conversation from our hostess, who sits back on her mattress, stately, watching proceedings.

He runs his hand through thick curly hair, talks about their house renovations, their son, as if he has no regard or too much regard for how he's being perceived.

He's not as good-looking as the other guy, but I'm drawn to him. I don't speak to him or look at him, hoping he'll notice me.

When he glances at me, I finally look over, and smile, and he smiles back, surprised.

Later, the hot tub beckons. We all cram in.

I ask about the neighbours – the house next door looks straight into the garden – a dark square of glass reflects sunlight and clouds.

The hostess shrugs. 'Let them look,' she says. 'Brighten up their boring lives.'

I wonder if this is what happens when you've been doing this for a while, if you become reckless, bold, walking out into traffic, not wearing a seat belt.

Gradually, people go inside, and I am left in the hot tub with the loud one. We're debating something that feels important. I have the strong feeling of holding my own, of words being mastered, of power. We pass the ball to each other, and I look in his eyes, and then look away.

'You're beautiful,' he says, his pupils dilating. 'I've wanted you from the beginning.'

This is what I want to hear, but it's not enough. I smile, but inside I think – is that all you've got?

I feel my jaws widening as if his head is inside and I could slowly, calmly, clamp down.

He kisses me.

Too soon, he reaches his hands under the water, his touch numbed and slippery by the flow. It feels strange, uncomfortable. I am too aware of the windows above us, of the smell of the chlorine, of his eyes, wanting something from me.

I should feel more, I think, so I climb on top of him, feeling my bikini top rise above the water, watching his eyes widen. I undo the clasp and take it off, unable to suffer fumbling fingers. I kiss him, grasping him in my hand. I hear him moan, gently, and I hold him slightly tighter.

I kiss him again, and try to lose myself.

I imagine I'm watching myself from the window upstairs and move accordingly.

I'm not sure how long we're out there, but when we come inside, everyone is busy.

I look for you from room to room. In a downstairs box room, I find the three women, piled on top of each other.

I call your name and your head emerges from the pile of bodies.

I smile at your grinning face.

'Just checking he's still alive,' I say, and everyone laughs.

'Join us,' someone says, but I shake my head.

'I need some water,' I say. 'But carry on.'

In the kitchen, I lean against the counter. The host emerges naked from the bathroom and checks something in the oven.

He pulls out a tray of canapés, of oven dim sum. 'Want some?'

I'm not hungry until I eat one, so I eat one more.

'Having fun?' he says.

'Too much,' I smile. 'I need a breather.'

In fact, I'm done.

The man from the hot tub returns while I am eating pizza, sitting on the edge of the sofa.

'Do you fancy finding a bed?' he says.

'I'm pretty tired,' I say.

He pouts, an oversized baby. 'Aw. I thought we were just getting started.'

'Sorry.' I hate myself for feeling bad.

He takes a canapé, chews it sullenly.

You come out from the bedroom, naked.

'You okay?' you say.

'I'm great,' I smile. 'There's food.'

You help yourself to a piece.

'I'm ready for round two,' the hot-tub man says to the room, but really to me.

His wife rolls her eyes. 'Give us a second, lover boy,' she says.

You come and sit beside me on the sofa. 'How are you feeling?' you ask, quietly.

'I'm ready for bed.'

You nod. 'Me too.'

Hot-tub man is talking again.

'I think we're going to head off,' I say.

He frowns. The host nods.

'So glad you guys could make it,' he says. 'We'll let you know if we do this again.'

In the car on the way home, you're buzzing, pregnant with the excitement of being wanted.

'All three of them took me by the hand,' you say, 'and dragged me off.'

You grin, and I see your path beside mine. I tell you about the hot tub, try to explain my disconnect.

'You like a challenge,' you say, but I'm not sure that's right.

The next day, we go wild camping at a place you've heard about. It's the first time we've left the business for more than one night: we have a new employee who comes each day to check people in, to reply to emails in a small office you've built. There's a thrill in driving away from it, but also a fear. I touch my phone in my pocket, telling myself not to check it. 'She'll call us,' you say, 'if she needs anything.'

We've packed the car with our old two-man tent, some essential clothes, flip-flops, insect repellent. We drive for a few hours and park on the outskirts of a small village we've never been to before. We follow a trail on your map, carrying our backpacks, our tents and sleeping bags: everything we will need. The trees are tall and ancient, arching overhead, the ground beneath them carpeted with ferns. As we walk further, the trail gets less defined and we see fewer people. I check myself, but my body still feels strong and ready to walk forever, despite the weight of my pack.

When you say, we come off the path and find a spot in a clearing on the shore of a beautiful broad loch. The surface is so flat and still; far out, I can see some moorhens gliding, but otherwise we are completely alone. We set up the tent under the trees and slide our bags inside. Without speaking, we slip off our clothes and run into the water. As the cold water washes over me, I feel the sweat of the walk, the drive, last night, melt away from my skin.

I float on my back, looking up at the sky, relishing the stillness of my mind. I know you are somewhere close by but I don't look for you.

I let my mind think about last night, about the man in the hot tub – why I didn't want him more.

Perhaps it was the setting: the lonely hot tub, the dying lawn.

I think of the tired Travelodge where we had our first threesome and know it can't be that.

I wanted him when he was separate to me, aloof, central to the group. He seemed bold and brave and I wanted to get close to him, to be alone with him. I wanted to make him see me, out of all the others, to choose me. I was pleased when we ended up in the hot tub together. I felt powerful when we were talking, drawing each other out. Then he told me he wanted me, and it was as if the evening ended. I knew the answer. If he hadn't said those words aloud, there would have been space for me to prove myself. Without that, I lost interest, went through the motions. It was as if I'd been playing a game with him, and when I saw I was going to win, the game was over.

I am learning so many things about myself: it is addictive, and I feel as if I'm only just scratching the surface.

*

Later, we build a fire with fallen wood. We cook dinner, enjoying the sounds of the birds, the dipping light of the long evening's sun. We sit together, peacefully, and we talk about all the things we've done. We work them out together. It's so wonderful to say aloud what is inside my head and have you listen with no ego, no judgement. Our conversations always feel like a collaboration.

We've had to learn this from having the business too: our different strengths have had to be pooled together. The hardest thing has been negotiating being a team when we have been used to working alone. We must communicate and form a plan together before acting. As we talk about this new sexual world we have entered, I realise we are doing the same thing here: figuring out how things work and why. We are helping each other, being completely together and completely separate at the exact same time.

When we are tired of talking, you get up and take off all your clothes. The sinking sun has turned the trees to silhouettes, the light on your skin is blue. You dance under the trees, taking my hand, pulling me up to join you. I defer, sitting on my log. There's something beautiful about watching you reach your potential, in your element. I know you are full of the joyful heat of being wanted, and I want that for you. You have spent so much of your life being ignored, unseen, that it is crucially important for you to be seen and valued now. I have given you that, but it's wonderful to see it starting up again for you, in this new world we've found.

It makes me want to find my own deep dark power, to understand it and to surrender.

Words

2019

One morning, I sit down at my desk. I push away invoices, the minutiae of a business life, and reach for the keyboard. The blank screen rises up. My fingers move as if propelled by something, and I watch the words appear on the screen.

They come out jarringly, in odd short lines, like poetry.

The first time, I'm afraid; of things falling into place, of knowing deeply that this is right.

It feels different this time, when the words come.

I must write them down.

If I don't catch them, they disperse to nothing, like smoke.

A few times, I think – I'll do it later – but when I look for them, they're gone.

The things I write are not to be seen.

They are for me, and perhaps for you, though I never show you. I write things I wouldn't say out loud; I'm honest in a way I couldn't be if I knew someone might read them.

I sketch out scenes we've acted out, and feelings that came with them.

I write about us, too. About the beginning of us. About her, before you. I try to do justice to how each moment felt.

Mostly I write about me, puzzling out things I have spent years wondering about.

I capture these things in a jar, not stopping to make sense of them.

I try to understand what we're doing.

I think about it, often.

I look for images in the world around us, in books and films. There is nothing that rings true to my experience: I find cautionary tales, broken marriages, lost causes.

If anyone mentions anything remotely sexual when we are out for dinner with friends, my attention rises, my throat burns. I push the conversation forwards. I drop sexual asides, hoping someone will be curious and pick them up.

I long to hear someone say – *I felt like that too.*

We don't tell anyone what we've been doing. It remains a precious secret between us.

Sometimes, I think about telling my closest friends, but I'm not sure how I would explain it, what words I would use. I don't understand it myself.

We talk about it, marvel at it.

I feel like we have crossed over some invisible,

understood line, and we are looking back at everyone we know, in their conventional lives. The rules we have lived inside are not real. I'm not sure it's possible for us to go back, even if I wanted to.

There is solace in the people we meet. We go for dinner with people who do what we do, and we automatically have something in common.

This is a social thing, more than a sex thing. The sex is part of it, but not the whole.

I have found the answer to the question I thought I wanted to answer.

I like women.

Like so much else, this is not the ending I expected it to be. There are still more things I want the answer to. Perhaps I am learning that there is no destination.

Holiday

2019

We meet them in a club in London. Our first time there, hidden in plain sight on a wide road near Liverpool Street. Inside, it's early and the place is empty. We explore the floors of nooks and crannies, a dungeon, themed rooms. I admire the creativity of the Headmaster's Office but am not yet ready for it.

Everything is wipe-clean and I feel uneasy. In this moment, fully clothed, I don't want to think about the rawness of sex, about what happens later. Pressure rises, which makes me turn away.

We grab a drink and take a seat on a mezzanine where we can watch the place fill out. We play a game of guessing people's jobs in their ordinary lives, what brought them here.

The eye contact as people pass becomes longer, more intense. Everyone seems hungry, blatant. We're not drawn to any of them, and I wonder if it's the location, the atmosphere, as much as the clientele. I start to feel the heavy drag of pressure: to choose someone, to make the night worth it. I look in your eyes and there is a question there but I can't make myself want them.

It's impossible to tell, until you know. We are about to leave, to give up, when we spot them. In the middle of the room below. There's something about the way they stand, the way he leans in to whisper in her ear that makes me think – maybe.

We strike up conversation. They're funny, normal, confident. We laugh, have things in common, feel them want us too. They tell us they are flying to Ibiza in the morning, and I think that's cool. We joke we will come too.

The music's loud: we can't quite hear each other. Someone suggests finding somewhere quieter, and we do, finding a cramped corner, joking about the ambience. We don't have sex, just touch and laugh and leave each other wanting more. The place isn't any sexier, but I care less now that they're here.

A few days later, she messages to invite us to Ibiza, half-joking. It's a quiet month. So we accept.

The lobby is marble-clean. I am wearing white shorts and feel fresh. We check in, drop the bags in our room. I step onto the balcony as the sun sets over the swimming pool, the ocean beyond.

'Nice hotel,' I say, as you put your arms around me.

'They have good taste.'

We shower and change, appraising each other. You – white linen shirt, blue shorts. Me – black skirt, chainmail top. We've been working out, running up the hill behind our house, lifting weights in our garage.

I've never found better motivation than being naked in a room full of strangers.

We walk through the streets to the pin they've sent us – a hotel where once celebrities partied, with a courtyard, swimming pool, palm trees. We take the lift to the top floor: a rooftop restaurant. It's quiet, a smattering of tables half full.

I'm wondering if we'll recognise them when I spot her. Dark hair, the glow of the day's sun on her face. She's wearing a white dress. He's sat beside her, hand resting on her knee, face crinkled in laughter. Brown hair, the stiff-necked look of a gym-goer.

We approach the table and they stand up. We kiss.

'We can't believe you're here,' she says.

You and I eat breakfast on the outdoor terrace, overlooking the sea. The sun is warm on my face; I close my eyes and feel it soak my skin. We take it in turns to go to the buffet: fruit course, egg course, pain au chocolat. The day spreads before us with only ourselves to think about. Coming here feels like a gift we've given to ourselves.

We walk to the old town. The streets are hot, and we climb steps to a lookout over the cobbled city.

We're meeting them in the lobby. Getting ready, I look at myself in the mirror and wonder if I'm good enough. She is shiny dark hair, no makeup, freckles, bright eyes. She has muscles where I don't. He's muscular too, but when I think of who I'm trying to impress, it's her.

When they walk towards us, I stand up tall, determined to fill this role. To be like them to an outside observer. You look great, beautiful, so I must too.

We hug, walking towards the car they've rented.

'Where are we going?' you ask.

'You'll see,' she says.

Looking out of the window, it feels wonderful to be taken care of. They must like us, I think, if they've gone to all this effort.

As we drive through the island's winding roads, the sea revealing itself at every bend under the startling sun, I feel free, happy, to be here now.

We turn the music up loud, talking shit, laughing. We tell our usual stories, spinning simple phrases we know are impressive, an elaborate sales pitch. *He was dating my flatmate. We used to live in Australia. He was like Indiana Jones. She's working on a book.* We take it in turns to big the other one up. We talk about the cottages. Our new-found, growing freedom. Our renovation of a barn to open a wedding venue.

They tell us their stories too, dropping details which are code words for desirability. He implies that she's from a rich family: her father is a prominent businessman. Where they live is an advertisement for wealth. They've recently applied for planning permission for an extension. She runs her own design business. He has his own gym. They act nonchalant, unimpressed by our achievements, and we do the same in return. We both behave as if work is a hobby, something we want rather than need, knowing this to be a trick: without necessity there is rarely success. We play an alpha game, and we're well-matched, which makes winning more precious, something I want.

We head downhill towards a beach, pulling into a small car park.

They glance at each other. He nods. 'I'll go and get a ticket,' he says.

On the beach, we find a man renting boats and choose one big enough for four.

The water is flat, the waves gently lapping the dock, the sea stretching to the cliffs and beyond. He helps me into the boat, his hand softer and warmer than yours.

You let him take the controls first; the engine revs and we zip out of the bay in the direction of the rocks. We're moving fast; I close my eyes and feel the forward momentum, the wind in my hair, the mist of salt water on my skin, the heat of the sun on my cheeks. I love this feeling of being moved, with no effort.

He offers to teach me to drive and I oblige, clambering into the front seat, listening to his instructions. When I move the hand throttle and the boat moves, I scream. 'Faster,' he says. 'Ride on top of the waves.' I steel myself, and push the stick forwards. It's thrilling, overwhelming. I long to be a passenger again.

He takes over, slowing down as we leave the bay itself, moving along the edges of the cliffs. There are fewer boats as we move further away. I feel my body on the smooth white seat. I look across at her. The wind is moving her hair back, her lips are slightly open. I imagine kissing her. I want to put my hand out and touch her arm.

The boat is slowing now. We pull into a sea cave with a small gravel beach and he looks back at her; they nod.

'Have you been here before?' I ask.

'We might have done a recce,' she says.

'For us?' I ask.

He shrugs.

I feel a rush of affection that they have considered us, their own desires on their holiday shifted to one side.

When the boat stops, we are moored on the sand at the back of the deep cave. The entrance, behind us, is lit up with an arch of daylight. Out there, somewhere, people are going about their days.

There is the sound of the waves lapping the shore, and then a splash as she jumps in, re-emerges, seal-like, her hair slicked back, smile white. You are already in the water, so I follow. Pulling my head up, you are all laughing, and I laugh too, the surprise of the water pulling me back to my body, my legs moving heavily underneath me, my breasts rising.

The echo in the cave is loud, bringing our laughter back to us as we lark about, splashing and play-dunking each other. You chase her across the space, water rising around you, and I hear her shriek as she is caught.

He has climbed back onto the boat and gestures for me to follow him. I swim back, aware of the moments stretching as he waits for me. He pulls me up out of the water. I am impressed by his strength, and when he kisses me, I find myself drawn to him: his tight broad chest, his muscular arms. I trace my fingers down his arms, across his body, dropping to my knees and looking up at him as I move down to his torso.

It is easy to admire him, so I do. I reach his shorts and feel him press his hips forward. I put my hands on his ass and pull him towards me. I take him out, moving my mouth and head rhythmically until he's pressed inside my throat. I look up at him. He is hard and I continue, faster, until he moans then takes my shoulders, pulling me up towards him, kissing me roughly on the mouth.

He leads me towards the front of the boat, where he can lay me back. Kneeling between my legs, he uses his tongue. I hold his head and move against him, wondering if I've ever done that with you. Turning my head to the side, I can see the other boats pass, and I wonder if they can see me. *Let them look*, I think, sinking below the surface.

He rises above me, his pupils wide, his lashes blinking water in the dim light. He finds a condom and rolls it on.

'Is this okay?' he says.

I nod, putting my hands above my head, ready for him as he enters me. He puts his hand over mine, holding me supine as he fucks me. The cove is upside down. He's gentle, strong, and when I look up, I feel a rush of affection for him, and reach my hands up, to pull him closer. We meld together and I lose time.

The sounds I make echo around the stone walls, bouncing towards you, out of the mouth of the cave.

I feel the power of being extraordinary, in broad daylight. I smile and float away.

We return the boat and lie on the beach in the sun, applying each other's sun cream, taking every excuse to touch.

I still have a slight feeling of wanting to impress them. Despite the effort with the cove, the moments I've shared with him. It is intoxicating, the not knowing.

He asks me what my fantasies are.

Even after everything, I'm not sure how to answer, and feel their eyes on me.

If I was the type to blush, I would.

'She likes to be the centre of attention,' you say.

Do I? I think.

I like to be lost in the moment. I try to explain, but can't find the words.

That night, we go for dinner in the old town.

We walk through the narrow streets, arm in arm, swapping partners. One moment, I walk with you, the next with him.

At the restaurant, we take turns being outrageous.

You dare her to remove her underwear and put it on the table, so she does. He sits beside me, stroking further and further up my thigh, while conducting a normal conversation. I burn, looking around the restaurant at the other couples, eating sedately in their holiday finery.

Smooth polpo slides down my throat. We eat garlic bread and joke about the taste, later. The sun fades behind us, and we order after-dinner drinks, chink them together and smile.

On the way back to the hotel in the taxi, it's her who strokes my leg. I feel an electricity as I look at her, wide-eyed, and meet her calm stare. She nods, infinitesimally, as if to say, *I want this, I want you.*

We go to our hotel room, which has a balcony, a view of the sea. I pull back the double doors, and she and I go outside, where it's quiet and the waves lap. Standing beside her, our hands touching on the balcony rail, I stroke my finger along hers. I look at her: our eyes meet, and I close the gap between us and kiss her. I feel her grasp onto me.

'Looks like you've started without us.' His voice is behind us, still inside. I smile, but don't break away from her. We've become a show, a spectacle, and I don't want this. I want her. I take her shoulders, moving my mouth away from hers, down her body. When I reach her waist, I drop to my knees, pushing her legs apart so she's standing, looking out to sea, her hands still on the balcony balustrade. From behind I lift her dress, pull her underwear aside, and use my tongue there, feeling her legs tremble, her back arch, with the movements I make.

'That's hot,' he says, but his voice is far away now, unimportant.

The next morning, they sleep in. We get up early, eat breakfast in the sun, relishing the moments alone. It's September, and the long winter will be beginning when we return home.

We message them but they don't reply.

We have plans to go to a beach club, but they've booked it and we don't know the timings. We take our things to the poolside, lie in the sun. The hotel is quiet, soft music plays. I read, you scroll your phone. We are both tense, full of the limbo of someone else's silence.

Eventually, they message, apologise. Tell us they will meet us at the pool.

When they arrive, they look tired behind their sunglasses. They ask if we're ready to go. We gather up our things and take a taxi.

We drive narrow, dusty streets. Crammed in the back of the cab, she looks out of the window. There is a gap between us, and I try to look at her, to smile, but she keeps her eyes outside.

When we arrive, we're shown to the day bed they've booked. We all cram on, applying our own sun cream, ordering drinks, joking about our hangovers. He's keen to get a package deal involving a bottle of spirits, mixers. We all agree, although my head is tight, my stomach hollow, my mouth dry. I want something to pick up the mood.

I read my book. The music is obnoxiously loud, designed for ravers, party animals. We are not that today. They lie close to each other. He seems quiet, sipping his drink, looking out to sea.

You suggest a walk on the beach, and I comply.

When we're far enough away, we talk.

'Are you picking up on something?' you say.

I nod. 'Perhaps they had an argument.'

We walk along the sand. 'I wonder if we did something wrong,' one of us says. We overanalyse, go through the events the night before. Everything seemed fun, light, easy.

'It's quite intense,' you say. 'Perhaps they need more space. It is their holiday after all.'

We come up with a plan, to do our own thing, to keep ourselves aloof.

We have a booking for lunch together in the restaurant on site. We have the usual conversations about home, about the gym, about our lives, but this time, it's as if the momentum has stopped. There's no subtext pulling things forward, and the conversation grinds.

I sip sangria, enjoy the sun, the food. Of course, their withdrawal makes me want them more, but I am adept at hiding that.

We lie and nap and drink and sunbathe. Then we return, get ready for a dinner booked in town.

As we shower, dress again, we ruminate. What could have changed? We wonder if we're imagining things: perhaps they're tired and that is all it is.

At dinner, things are still awkward. On the same streets we laughed along last night, we walk sedately with our own partners. No games, no dares to liven up the meal. We eat, talk of the long day, how we're tired. They tell us of their plans to drink less, train more when we've gone home, and it feels their real holiday might begin.

Back at the hotel, we climb the lift together. You invite them to our room: they say they'll grab some stuff and be there soon. We lie in bed, watching foreign television, waiting, but they do not come. We talk it over every which way, trying to understand, to work out what is real and what we are imagining.

In the morning, we get up early to go to the airport. We send them a message, thanking them for an amazing time, and suggesting we'll see them again in the UK.

Nothing.

All the ticks on our messages are grey. We google this, convince ourselves we've been blocked. We spend most of the time in the airport, and in the air, wondering what happened.

We've been ghosted, we say to each other, using a term for single people younger than us.

When we get back, home seems dull and grey compared to the sunlit fantasy of Ibiza. The memories, though good, are tainted with whatever happened after. We are investigating the scene of a crime we're not sure took place. We go over and over details and facts, and it's like we're worrying a loose tooth that will never come out.

We hold each other close in bed that night, our bruised egos dulled by the presence and love of each other. Imagine if we were single, we say to each other. How hard this would be alone. I think of my best friend, before she met her husband. How she was repeatedly rejected. I have an insight into how that must have felt, and want to message her. But she doesn't know yet what we've been doing. I know I will tell her, I'm just not sure how. How hard it would be to explain. So much has happened; we have drifted so far off shore.

'How was your holiday?' people ask, on our return.
How do I begin to answer?

Stop

2020

Inside this barn, years of labour, work and thought sit.

The stone walls, smoothed and repointed, look anew. We've planned the lighting to mimic candlelight, to throw warm yellow and white to highlight grooves and age. Hanging from the high, beamed ceiling: an iron chandelier, ready to drip with eucalyptus foliage. We've planted olive trees in giant pots and placed them about the room.

Huge wooden doors took work to sand and oil. They had to come off their hinges, be put back on. It took a team of ten to lift them into place.

When I stand inside it now, switch on the lights, the barn lies empty. Rows of cross-backed chairs face the front, await the witnesses.

We've been rushing to a deadline, painting final bits, installing everything we'll need. We have bookings, spread across the spring and summer.

But overnight, everything has changed. The world has stopped in its tracks, told to stay at home, indoors.

Last night, we stayed up late, sitting around the kitchen table, making our Plan B.

I'm frustrated, angry: we've worked on this for three years, secured the money, permissions, and now it all must wait.

I'm scared too: we have a loan to pay off, and staff ready to start work. We must call all those with bookings and rearrange.

You are calm, as if you've been waiting for a crisis all your life. Despite the lack of information, the panic all around, you sit still and think. I try to talk things through, but you are gone inside your head.

The next day, the phone is ringing off the hook: bookings at the cottages wanting money back, people asking to postpone their big days. We put the new team to work, answering phones, collating information, updating our rudimentary website. We move as fast as we can, but there aren't enough hours in the day.

There is no time for writing.

Everything is on hold, but also moving fast. We're busy, managing a larger team, working out the answers moment by moment as things change. You and I think fast, to keep the money flowing in. We set up a website to do local deliveries, working with our new wedding suppliers, pulling strings to find produce, flour, bread. Orders flood in: the team we have employed for other tasks take to the road, packing boxes in the empty barn until late at night.

The days and weeks spin by: the barn waits, and we fill our time with more pressing concerns.

Our other life is on hold too. We're back at the beginning again: our minds and bodies full, no time for thinking about anything else. We fall into bed. But this time, no matter how tired we are, our bodies touch.

By being restricted, we learn that we value freedom.

We find pockets of it in this new world, but we don't like rules.

A bright clear day, we drive to the lake after work. A new sign, stuck at an angle. No swimming: deep water.

Twigs crunch underfoot as we traverse the woodland path – it is the time of year for bluebells, and there is a carpet of them beneath the trees. I grab your arm, to stop us and take it in – the dappled sunlight of the early evening, the beginnings of the long summer ahead.

We reach the water's edge, pull off our clothes, dropping them onto a low tree branch. We wade into the cold water, and I tell myself – as I always do – that these chilly first steps are always worth the feeling of deep calm we find, floating in the circle of dark water, surrounded by only dense trees, the swift movement of birds, and the broad expanse of the sky.

Cloaks

2020

When we hear about the party, we can't believe it's real. The world is opening up, but still. We book tickets anyway, hoping for it to be true.

A country pub in a stone village. We carry our finery through the diners, my cloak swathed in a dry-cleaning carrier. We have a room at the back, overlooking a windy street of small houses.

We walk through the town to a palace. It almost feels normal, as people go about their days: walking dogs, yoga mat slung over one shoulder, dog lead in one hand, flat white in another. We still give each other a wide berth on the pavements. We pop into the deli and buy sausage rolls and potato salad, waiting in line in masks for takeaway cappuccino. Sitting on the grass with a grand facade behind us, we eat our picnic.

It's summer, and the air is almost warm. Closing my eyes, I feel myself smile.

The dress code is black lingerie for the women with long black capes, masks, nothing else. Black tie for the men. We take photos of ourselves reflected in the brass mirror on the wall in the hotel room: smiling, pouting, me kissing your cheek.

As I apply my makeup in the bathroom mirror, I wonder what the night will bring. I have the same feeling I had when we'd go out when we were teenagers, at university, the delicious excitement that anything might happen. I'm excited about seeing someone across the room, wanting them. Perhaps I will find myself brave enough to pursue them.

We drive to the venue – a stately home, lit with flames. I imagine the clattering of horses' hooves on cobbles, long dresses, corsets, bonnets.

We pass the dark-panelled doorway, and are checked in. Inside is busy. The people who run these parties do it secretly: you have to know about them. You have to have a password, a code. They attract models, actors, people with power. I'm drawn to these people, confident in their bodies, in their minds. We joke about how it makes me shallow. You prefer the less pretentious parties, with friendlier people. I need a barrier to want somebody.

Outside in the garden, crowds gather around statues, topiary. We wear masks on our faces but not our mouths.

How did they get away with this? people ask each other.

Someone tells us they told the council it was a wedding. Earlier in the day, there had been a woman in a wedding dress photographed in the garden. They have been asked to keep the party outside, and none of us is sure that will be possible. Someone says there is a pool, but no one can find it amongst the grounds.

It's the buzz of the party that none of us should be here at all.

We explore the house with our drinks in hand. Upstairs is cordoned off, but we duck under the red rope. We find the bedrooms, empty now, the places where things will happen later.

Back downstairs, you find the toilets. I wait for you in the lobby. I'm examining some of the portraits on the walls when I see him. Standing, broad in his tuxedo, rocking on his heels, holding a woman's handbag. Dark hair, face creased lightly from smiling.

We catch eyes, and he smiles at me, looks away.

Something about him makes me bold.

'Waiting for someone?' I ask. He looks at me properly. 'The handbag,' I say. 'I assume it isn't yours.'

He looks down at the ball of sequins he's holding, and smiles. 'I forgot I had this.'

A slight accent.

'Where are you from?'

'Poland.'

'That's a long way to come.'

'We live in London now. We'll travel for this.' He gestures around the empty panelled lobby, towards the double doors where we can see the edges of the party.

She comes out of the toilets, walks towards us. Her black lingerie is the expensive sort, and her body is perfection. She has long red-brown hair, a china doll face. She smiles at me, warily.

He kisses her cheek. 'We just met,' he says. 'This is –'

I introduce myself, holding out my hand formally.

She takes it, shakes lightly.

I don't remember what we talk about.

I remember fishing, casting a line and attempting to catch a bite. I want to say the right things to draw them towards me. She's beautiful, but this time, it's him I'm drawn to.

As we talk of ordinary things, there's a space between us wide enough for want to spread. The conversation feels balanced, equal.

I want this to lead somewhere.

It isn't the usual feeling of being pulled along by a tide. I want to walk on water.

After a while, we decide to explore.

We go up to the playroom, which is now awash with bodies, blowing off the steam of the last few months. It's dark, red-lit, and the mass of moving naked people is something difficult to watch but also difficult to look away from.

There's little room in here and it's hot, sweaty.

I imagine stepping inside, trying to find room for us four. Looking for a gap, having to fight for space. It doesn't feel right to me.

I turn to you. 'This is a bit much for me,' I say.

You nod.

'I think perhaps we'll go.'

You look at them.

'I know,' I say. 'I like them too, but this . . .' I gesture at the room. 'It isn't how this should be.' I know this is a risk. But for the first time, I back myself and us.

'I think we're going to go,' I whisper to her. 'It's so busy in here. It doesn't feel sexy to me.'

Saying what I really feel is like jumping into cold water.

'I was just thinking the same thing.' She pauses. 'We have a place. We could all go there. Let me speak to him.'

She moves across the room. I watch them talk. I feel in some way this is a step for her, as it is for me. A mutual movement towards what we want.

We all agree to meet at their place. I have the address on a piece of paper. As we queue to retrieve our coats, I wonder if we'll lose our steam. But before we leave, we swap numbers and she squeezes my hand. 'You'll come, won't you?' she says. I squeeze back, and nod.

They only have one bottle of wine, are apologetic, as if they are used to providing better. We shrug, and I want to laugh. I don't care about the wine.

We share it out and sit around and chat. The flat is small, with an open-plan living area, a small kitchen, one bedroom. We talk of lives far from here, of what we have in common.

It's always hard to remember the way things start,

impossible to pinpoint the moment when all the tensions in the room reach the right pitch for someone to act.

    She's touching you; you are kissing.

    I reach forward and kiss him. I feel his stubble with my fingers, holding his hand in mine, moving my other hand down his body. I can feel the heat of his want, but I can also feel part of his focus on her, on you. His mind is here, with me, but also with her, and there is something respectful about his care that makes me want him more.

    I climb on top of him on the sofa and he takes off my clothes. He looks at my body like he is pulling back a curtain on an amazing view. I glow inside. In an instant, I see his focus shift wholly onto me, away from her. It turns me on: I take his hand and put it inside my underwear. His eyes wide: I move on his fingers, tipping my head backwards, making noises. Part of me hopes that she can hear, that you can. I kiss him, deeply, wanting him to lose himself in me.

    Keeping his fingers on me, he tips me off his lap onto the sofa. He's gentle, but he's also firm as he kisses down my body. I tilt my nipples into his mouth and feel his tongue flick; my eyes roll. When he stops between my thighs, I'm ready, open. He pulls aside my underwear and slowly rubs his tongue down there. The darkness behind my closed lids goes white; I hear noises that must be mine. I am finally inside.

Bright Lights

2020

It is a city I know, but can't navigate well. Sharp glass fronts beside the sandstone facades. The brick, still traced with old soot, names marked out, businesses long gone.

We've booked a suite in a 1920s-style hotel, with a rooftop bar and restaurant. We walk through the city, relishing our new freedom. I try on expensive lingerie, dressing up for you in various colours while you flirt with the attractive salesgirl. Wanting to impress her and myself, I try on bondage-style outfits, leather look, with heavy metal clasps which push my breasts together. I pull back the curtain of the changing room boldly. I like the way I look in them, an evolved version of myself. I feel ready to take control, to wield a whip.

That night, we walk to their apartment, where there is a doorman in a suit. I'm polite, as if he might say no, you can't come in.

We climb high in the lift and he welcomes us at the door, a shiny suit, slicked hair, smelling of new things: car leather, cologne. She wears a flowery top and mini skirt, is bending to pull on red-soled heels, leather with two straps across her ankle.

He opens glass doors and proudly lets the city in, the broad horizon dazzled with lights. I step out onto the narrow balcony, looking down at the vehicles snailing below. The long drop makes my mind whirl. I look for landmarks, but in the darkness all the lights look the same.

You hand me a cocktail in a tumbler, sharp and lemony, and I step back inside.

His voice is coarse like pebbles rolling on the sand. He loudly tells us of his life; she nods and smiles beside him. I ask how long they've lived here.

'Seven years,' he says.

'I've been here three,' she says.

'It's such an amazing place,' I say, and watch him smile.

We go out to eat, taking a taxi as heeled women shouldn't have to walk.

The restaurant is dressed up with fake foliage, running up the wall outside, continuing through the entrance door. I think of fairy tales, a house at the top of a beanstalk. Women on stilts throw fire and gyrate in the golden light.

We're still getting used to being free again, being out. The world feels as if it could close up again at any moment, like a clam, and we hold on to it.

We're led to a table inside by someone beautiful.

Handed menus, but he orders for us all. She excuses herself for a cigarette, and I follow her down the stairs.

'How did you meet?' I ask, inhaling, watching others walk by.

'At work,' she says. 'He's such a gentleman.' She pauses, takes a drag. 'It's amazing to find a man who offers all this.'

She gestures at the restaurant, the street, as if he is the keeper of the city.

I nod, and think of you and me. I want to offer things to myself.

'I haven't always been treated this well,' she says, and I lean in, despite myself. But she stops there, stubs out her cigarette, and we go inside.

The food comes out on tiny plates and we assume this means it's good.

We talk and laugh; he rolls the conversation on. We all join in, and somehow the evening is easy, flies by.

After food, we return to theirs, where the city still sparkles. We are told to change into lingerie while they make drinks. In their bedroom, I'm excited to try on my new things, and she is complimentary, admiring me. I smile inside.

She chooses something similar from a huge array she lays out on the bed. We both look like extras from a porn film, and laugh about it, downing cocktails for courage before we emerge.

His eyes flick over us as we come out and he smiles.

Later, when we're all at play, he puts a hand around her throat. She makes a noise and you and I glance at each other.

Drink makes the moments blur. I'm on the bed with him and you're beside me, with her. You're on top and she has her legs in the air, her hands above her head. She's writhing, moaning, both wanting and not wanting more.

He's on top of me, touching me. His fingers move inside too quickly, and I feel my walls go up. When he kisses me, he moves his tongue fast, as if speed means passion. It feels as if he's playing a game of tennis without a partner, against a wall. I close my eyes, and wait for it to end.

I feel fingers there again, between my legs. When I open my eyes, it isn't fingers but his dick, moving unsheathed inside my body. His eyes are looking at my tits, unfocused, and he's making noises that sound fake, like something he has heard in porn.

I feel sick but do not move.

I glance across at you, still absorbed with her. I close my eyes, let it happen. Next time I open them, he has pulled out; something white is on my leg.

I get up and go to the bathroom, sinking against the door. In the mirror, I see a whore, with bleary, smudgy eyes and slutty lingerie. Inside, I'm hollow, can't examine how I feel.

When I emerge, you're with them, lying on the bed. I join you, but can't speak as you make small talk. You look at me, and know there's something wrong, and so we leave.

We can't talk in the taxi with the driver there, so watch the city pass. I try to think whether what happened was wrong or not. It feels wrong, but how do I explain?

When we're alone, I tell you what has happened. I say the words *he fucked me without a condom*. I explain the things around it, but this is the headline.

I shower for a long time in our fancy hotel room.

When I emerge, you put your arms around me, ask me why I didn't say anything.

I don't know how to answer.

You look into my eyes. 'If you'd said something, I –' you stop.

You'd what? I want to say. 'I didn't know how. It seemed pointless to ruin everyone's fun. What was done was done.'

'You need to say something if you're not comfortable.'

'It's not that easy.'

'If we're going to do this, it has to be. You have to speak up for yourself. I can't always be watching you, checking on you.'

You hold me in the bed as we fall asleep. I can tell you feel bad, as if this is your fault.

Part of me thinks it is, but knows it's not. I want to be my own person, strong, alongside you. I want us to be equals.

Lying in the dark hotel room, I feel alone, despite

you being there. I try to understand why I didn't push him away, or say anything. What words would I have used? There's no word for what he was doing – it wasn't rape; I wanted to be there, to have sex with him. But he was willing to put me at risk for his own pleasure, as if not asking was part of the thrill for him. He was getting off on taking something from me. That was the violation.

Sometimes, crossing roads makes us realise where we're safe. We learn to hold our hands up when a truck comes fast and stop traffic.

This is how we learn the edges of our yes and no.

Out

2021

We go to visit my oldest friend. We haven't seen each other since before the pandemic, and so much has happened, I'm worried we'll never catch up.

Her daughter is walking now, stumbling across the kitchen, bringing us toys and books while we drink tea and talk. You and her husband are outside, building a fence for their new chickens.

'What's new with you?' she asks, and I don't know where to start.

'We had a threesome,' I blurt out. As soon as the words are out in the kitchen, I regret them.

She is open-mouthed. I try to explain, in a few sentences, what has led to this. Trying for a baby, loss of sex drive. The business, achieving things, power. There is no satisfactory way of putting this into words, even to myself.

'I'd always wondered if I liked women,' I say, finally.

These words sit between us, said aloud at last.

I know she has been with women too: years ago, she got drunk with one of our school friends and they went down on each other. I wonder if she'll say *me too*, but she doesn't.

'What was it like?' she says.

'Good,' I say. I feel again the inadequacy of language.

She asks practical questions. Where did we meet? How did we choose? What were the conversations, before and after?

'Were you not afraid of seeing him with someone else?' she asks.

'Of course,' I say. I try to explain that too.

She says she understands. She talks of experimenting when she was single – because we met so young, we never really had that. I tell her about the parties, the glamour, the buzz of being wanted. She says it sounds like fun.

She asks if she can tell her husband and I say yes, but only him.

'Did you tell her?' you ask later, when we're going to bed.

I nod. 'She understood.'

It feels strange to have told someone. Strange, but also thrilling.

We lead a double life. We run the business: managing the team, checking the books, going to yoga classes, meeting vanilla friends for dinner.

I run along the river, feeling the fresh air rush past, learning the strength of my new body.

We hold meetings, are sensible, do what is necessary.

We attend family meals, buy birthday presents, pay bills.

The other part of our lives is lived below the surface. We take mini-breaks to London, where we get dressed up and fuck new friends in glamourous, soft-lit places. We go out for dinner, drinks, with people met online. Each new night brings the tension of what we will find, and whether we will like it.

Centre

2021

The table is laden when we arrive: platters of glistening perfect sushi, cut fruit in various intricate shapes. It has been pushed to the side of the room, leaving the wooden floors clear. Between two tall bay windows is a large black frame in the shape of a cross.

Our hostess is cover-girl perfect. Expensive lingerie: black with gold accents; red hair, clear blue eyes. Her features combine in a way that makes it hard to look directly at her.

Her hand shakes as she pours champagne. They fascinate me, these small vulnerabilities that expose the very beautiful, the very rich, the very glamorous. The greatest thrill is to walk amongst these people and be accepted by them – I am always looking for cracks.

The other guests arrive: a famous model who is now a DJ. He tells me he grew tired of surface, of being seen, and longed to give something, to create. Inside, I think – how shallow. But I do what I am good at, what I've always done, reflecting his best light back at him. I hold the reins and pull down, watching them take.

*

We are offered a small white pill on a silver tray. You decline, chivalrously. I take it onto my tongue and swallow. I think of urban legends, of warning videos shown in dimmed classrooms. I imagine my throat closing in.

I wait for something to happen, checking myself for changes. I watch the lights blur, and I wonder – is this how I'm supposed to feel?

There is a girl who wears long black patent boots, laced up, shiny. I am mesmerised. I ask to try them on and she unravels the long laces, pulls them off. I feel my toes constrict. She eases them over my thighs gently, pulling tight. I close my eyes and smile and kiss her.

She is wearing the boots again now, impossibly high. She stands tall in the centre of the room, next to a black frame, a giantess, Amazonian.

I step forwards, in my underwear. I feel eyes on me. I feel myself turn under their gaze. I don't worry about how bright my light is, how it might be too much. I only do, I only am.

She turns my back to the watching room, placing my hands on the frame, arms prostrate. Automatically, I lean forwards and am exposed.

Bend over, she whispers, arch your back.

She stands in front of my face then, leans down and speaks softly so the others cannot hear. Her eyes are cat-green, clear. She tells me to be calm. She counts my breaths, in and out, in and out.

Be in your body, she says, now. Feel it, here.

She puts her hand on my chest.

I close my eyes and breathe. Air fills my lungs and I feel my bra expand along my rib cage, my nipples pressing mesh. I feel a beat between my legs. Spreading, upwards, through, around.

She strokes my buttocks with something soft but firm. A long leather whip with many ends. Caress, I think. More.

You are safe, she says. Give me a number, between one and ten.

I don't understand, until I feel the gentle slap of the whip across my skin.

Two, I say, wanting more.

There is a maddening pause, a rubbing of the smooth black on my skin. Then, again, a slap. Harder this time, a tingle spreads.

Four, I say.

I want to impress those in the room, but push those thoughts away. I am here, now, I think.

This time, the slap clacks. I feel impressed, fear, want.

Six, I say. I long to see how much I'll take.

She rubs for longer, gentle, teasing. I bite my lip, arch back, lift onto tiptoes.

Woah. A shooting pain, and then the tingle. Feeling cascades; I close my eyes and long for touch between my legs.

Nine, I say.

More? she whispers.

Yes.

This time, my mind goes blank. Delicious, clear, there's nothing there. Like being dunked in cold black water. I cease. The room is calm and still.

Breathe, I hear her say, and so I do.

I feel a tingling, spreading down my legs. I feel my heartbeat. I feel my breath, rising and falling around me. I feel the moment I am in rise up to meet me.

Later, I am spread out and people touch me. I open my body. I cry out. I am rising, rising, rising. I fill my own mind.

I am the centre: things move around me. It feels inevitable, like the answer to a question I didn't know I had been asking.

Wedding

2021

They stand at the front of the barn, silhouetted in golden lights. They turn to each other and say the words we all long to say. They promise to love each other, to support each other, to be faithful to each other.

I stand close to the back, out of sight, and watch. I see the chandelier bursting with fresh greenery, the lights aflame. I see one of our managers, in a suit, holding a clipboard in his hands. I see the tension around his temple as he listens to each word, waiting for the next cue, the next thing he needs to do to spin this golden day. I feel a rush of fondness, that he cares.

In high season, couples stand in this space and make these promises. It is not lost on me that we watch this, over and over, and then we break our own.

Your oldest friend comes to tell us he is leaving his wife.

At first, he gives us the cover story. He tells us they have been unhappy for a long time. He talks of marriage counselling, of love languages, of mismatches.

His voice, as he sips his tea at the kitchen table, is

squeaky clean. He talks too fast and too determinedly for the whole truth.

There is more, we both think, independently. We look at each other and we wait.

'It all got too much,' he says. 'I had to make a change. For me. For us.'

We nod, as if we believe him.

'So it was a mutual decision?' you ask.

'Yes,' he says.

I wish she was here, to contradict or agree. I long to hear her words, to see whether her story is the same.

It's not until dinner that he tells the truth. A glass of wine, face flushed. You ask something, and it all comes tumbling out.

The work colleague. The fumbled, melting kiss that changes everything. That solidifies his dissatisfaction into action. He has a reason now, a ship to jump to.

He has leaped quickly, seeing a new sunny place. The beginning of something. They reflect their own positive qualities back at each other. They are seen in the best light. It is easy for him to blame his past problems on the wrong partner, the wrong situation.

He thanks us for listening, for not judging him.

'All that matters is that you are happy,' you say.

He smiles wildly, brightly, with relief. 'I am,' he says. 'I really am.'

We whisper about it at night.

What do you think? we ask each other, over and over.

We are not certain he is really in love. It's easy to think that in the hot fire of the beginning. But who are we to say? And does it matter anyway?

We whisper our thoughts in case he can hear them from the spare room. We don't want to be the ones to bring him back to reality.

It's easy to be the ones on the outside, casting judgement. I remind myself that we do not have a conventional marriage. From the outside, we are dysfunctional too.

We have found a way to exist in reality together: to support each other and also let each other be free. We are like cats, we say to each other, we could be anywhere, but we choose to be here.

Are you worried I'll leave? you say, smiling.

You do leave, I say. But you always choose to come back.

Dinner

2021

You've found them online. There's preliminary work, sorting through potentials, curating our profile, where anonymous photos show parts of our bodies in good lighting. I'm not interested in specifics, in which photos are chosen and in what is written about us in some secret, accessible place online. You handle this and I am aware this is a gift given, a burden lifted.

You show me photos of potential meets and I say yes or no. In some ways, this makes me a gatekeeper, the final veto, the one who can undo all your hard work with just one word. It makes you selective. Often, the men are less attractive than the women – those ones do not make the cut. You know what type I like: tall, fit, nice smile. I'm not interested in seeing nudes, photographs of body parts. People only send face photos when there's trust built and these are the ones you show me.

We don't discuss it but there is a flimsy privilege in being able to choose, in being in demand. We are aware, vaguely, that it may not always be like this.

*

We meet them at a tapas bar in town. The music is reminiscent of holidays, though outside is unrelenting grey. We joke about the weather over sangria, cheersing to the curse of being British.

He's tall and jumpy, with slightly stooped shoulders, mouth held in an apologetic tilt. She's small with dark hair and an elfish grin. The type of person you'd imagine reading gothic romance.

As soon as I see them, I think: *No*. I'm not attracted to him. The way he talks too fast and won't meet my eye belies an insecurity which makes me turn away. They are obsessed with minutiae — where we will sit at the table; there is a moment where he gasps, thinking he has lost his phone. She overanalyses the menu, asking the waitress too many questions.

As we settle, order drinks, they speak about their lives in an overcompensatory way. It's like looking at something too familiar: there is no purchase, no mystery. I want to grasp them by the lapels, tell them to slow down, that they are pushing me away. How much easier it would be if I could just say *I'm not feeling this*. Try that. But this situation is not just about me. There are four people here: each one must find compatibility in the swamp of the unknown. It's like playing a game where you must roll a silver ball around until it fits in place. Attraction is strange and hard to quantify.

I glance at you to see if you are feeling the same, but you are laughing, leaning forward, and I think, *Oh no*.

I tell myself not to retract; to not judge them quickly or unfairly. I sit back in my seat and sip my drink, waiting for the moments I can shine. But they roll the conversation on and on. Occasionally, they ask us things, but every time I speak, she leans forward with a question mark upon her face, asks me to speak louder, as if I'm shy or softly spoken when I know I'm not. The restaurant is loud, buzzy. He teases her for being deaf, but it feels like a silencing, even if it's not. It makes me cease to try.

There's a barrier here, between me and them, and I wonder if you feel it too. It's annoying when this happens: the anticipatory moments that have led to this seem wasted now. The time we took to plan, get ready, escape our other commitments. The hopes of a lubricated evening flying on its own are dashed.

Usually, I love this part, over dinner and drinks, when we talk, enjoy nice food and feel the tension stretch elastic across the table. I love the build-up just as much as what happens later. This is the part when anything is possible, when all still exists in the ordinary world.

'So, how did you get into this?' I ask, thinking perhaps they will pique my interest. I'm always fascinated by the reasons people are drawn here, to do these things.

They smile, and I watch him reach for her, under the table.

There's a few ways this could go, and you can never

predict which it will be. Sometimes I think I have a couple worked out, but I'm often surprised.

For them, he has always fantasised about seeing her with another man. We've seen this one before, in variations. For some, it's about humiliation: about sitting in the corner of the room and not being able to join in. Wanting to be taunted, to feel their belly flip over, worst-case scenarios – that they are not good enough – rising up to meet them. For others, they want to be in control, to be the facilitator, the one who allows such things to happen. You can fuck my wife, but only because I say so.

For him and her, he wants to see her be sexual. He likes to see her lose control, to fall into the deepest places inside herself. He likes to witness it. Watching it happen with another man, someone who isn't him, heightens the pleasure of it.

The interesting thing about desire is that you can't take the person's word for why they like something. They can't take their own word either. So much of what we want is below the surface, out of our grasp. We feel something deep and visceral, and we explain it later. We want reasons for things when maybe there are none. The unknown is not a bad thing. But it is fascinating, drawing us in and under.

As I watch him talk of her desire, part of me wants to see it in action. Part of me wants to go to the next step just to witness it. But I know if we go there, I will have to be an active participant. This is not a field trip. And I don't want to see them without their clothes on – sometimes, it's just as simple as that.

Later, when the food is finished and we don't want more drinks, I feel a pressure rising.

He asks several times where we are staying, how far it is to home.

I glance at you, and you are looking back, a question mark between your eyes. I long to be alone with you to discuss what we both want. To tell you that I don't want them.

Several things coalesce inside my chest at once: an old tendency to make people happy, to push my own desire aside and go along, to take the path of least resistance. I could do this. I know I can make myself come, or make someone else do it. Simultaneously, I know I can't do it, that I don't want to. I imagine them, making noises, naked on a bed, and that image is what makes me speak.

'I'm not feeling great,' I say. 'I think I need to go to bed.'

They both blink at me across the table. The moment stretches loaded like thunderclouds massing on a sunny day and I feel deeply bad. Their faces drop, their shoulders sag. I'm not certain how much is my imagination, but I feel a visible heaviness descend, which could be my own guilt.

'Let's get the bill,' you say, and it's as simple, easy, as that.

On the way back to the car, and home, I feel relieved but also terrible. I ramble on at you, about desire and how I didn't feel it, intellectualising, muddying something obvious.

'I just didn't fancy them,' I say, finally.
I take a breath – that's it, that's all it is.
You nod. 'That's fine. You are allowed to say no.'
'I just feel bad. Would you have gone with them?'
You shrug. 'I would, I think.'
'Did you like them?'
'Not particularly.'
'So why then?'
'I think she was into me, and it would have felt good, to feel desired.'

I consider this: why him wanting me wasn't enough. We discuss it, as we have before. You like to be desired, to be seen, to be wanted. You want to be the architect of someone else's deepest pleasure, triggering them to act automatically, genuinely, stripped back to their core. It is an act of service that only you can orchestrate and this is what turns you on.

I also want to be desired, but not by anyone. I want the attention of the most unattainable person in the room. Either emotionally distant, self-contained, or the most in demand. The highest on the social pecking order. I want someone who knows their own mind to want me, to choose me.

'I'm sorry,' I say.

'Don't be,' you say. 'We can fuck instead.'

When we get home, we do. We come together with the thrill of being each other's person, of being in this together.

As I go to sleep, I feel bad for them, seeing their faces behind closed lids. But I also can't change the way I feel.

You/Me

2021

Sometimes, the night is about you, and sometimes me. Sometimes, there is equilibrium and balance.

There is no way to know before, when we are in our hotel room. When I am smoothing cream onto my face, lining my eyes, glancing at each angle until I glimmer, like an edited photograph. When you are shining shoes rarely worn and already complaining about the strictures of your tuxedo.

There is no way to know as we eat in a restaurant, sitting out on the street for the first time this year, soaking in the warm evening after a long, cold winter. I sit up straight, suck spaghetti through my lips, taste salt and cream and some unknown herb. You sip chilled white, leaving ghost fingerprints on the glass. I take your hand across the table and you take a photo.

There is no way to know as we wait in the queue outside the venue. Various ordinary addresses made extraordinary by what is happening out of sight. We make small talk, picking up tiny gestures like charms on a silver chain: a glint of eye contact, the curve of a smile. I wonder – will I choose you? Will this be the track this night will take?

There is no way to know as our tickets are scanned, as we sign NDAs and promise to behave.

Or as we change into underwear.

Even as the night thrums beneath our fingertips.

It is what makes it so exciting.

You:

Holding a woman high up on the frame of a four-poster bed. Brazilian, she brings to mind Victoria's Secret, long legs flashing along catwalks, cameras snapping. I am with her husband, rocking back and forth, fingers on my own clit. I bend and sway, and catching sight of you, I stop.

There is something sublime about my view: a feeling so large I struggle to take it all in. It is the same feeling as trying to capture something real and raw in words, on paper.

It is a sort of awe, of pride, of majesty.

It is a sense that one day, you will remember this. When we are old and tired, sitting on a veranda, in rocking chairs. You will turn to me and say, *Do you remember when* . . .

I will smile, eyes crinkling, nod, and reach out for your hand.

*

Me:

Reaching out for the hand of a girl I like, pulling her towards me and putting on a show.

It is me and her, dancing when we were young, drawing people in. It is standing on the edge of a swimming pool and diving into the cool, deep water. It is being wild and free.

Us:

Feeling the eyes of other women skirt our skin as we walk through the club. I feel their gaze and don't know if it's you or me or both, all at once.

We find a sofa and cradle drinks, taking in the things around us. People in a swimming pool, playing. This is an underground sauna, and we are in swimwear, mine bright under UV lights, making me glow.

Then they are there, before us. A crowd of five women, all beautiful, all different. One small and slight with dark hair, another blonde and brave: the one who speaks.

We think you're beautiful, they say.

I think of fairies, materialising in the gloom.

They take us each by the hand and lead us off to darker corners.

You:

Later, when I am spent, you take two of them to the pool and have them both at once.

I sit on a sofa and watch.

Do I feel abandoned, left out, lost?

No. I am satiated, full with the night. If I want more, it's there, waiting. All I need to do is reach out and take it.

It is like a pendulum swinging, to you and me and back again.

Model

2021

We invite friends for dinner and a life drawing class in the barn.

Your friend from childhood – bearded and barrel-chested – and his wife. They met at work on a bat survey: they're ecologists. I like them both; they're interesting and honest. Deeply passionate about the world around them. On long walks, they'll stop mid-sentence, hearing the sound of a rare bird, mating far away.

They don't know what we do.

They arrive early. I pour strong gin and tonics, and we cheers. They ask about the business. We ask about London, their cats.

He has invited one of his colleagues who lives nearby.

She walks into our kitchen – blonde, bold – apologising for being late.

Your friend introduces her.

'This is V,' he says. 'My friend from work.'

'Thanks for letting me crash the party,' she says, kissing you on both cheeks.

She leans in for me. She smells soapy clean.

*

The model stands in the centre of the circle of our chairs. She moves as she is told to. Her legs are slightly astride, one arm stretched above her head, the other at her waist.

I feel my stick of charcoal move across the page, sketching the outline of her body, the darkness between her legs. I let my mind go dull and flat, focusing on the way her long red hair falls over her shoulders.

When I look up, my eyes meet V's across the circle. She is looking past the model right at me. She smiles, turning away.

Once all the paying guests and the tutor have left, we cook together in our house. Your friend helps with the easy tasks: assembling salad in a bowl, chopping tomatoes, readying the steaks. We lay the table, light candles, turn the music up. V deftly uncorks a bottle of wine; I watch the muscles in her arms tighten as she pulls it free. We chink our glasses, drink.

We talk about how beautiful the model is. I feel the confidence of her words, and I wonder: perhaps she likes women too.

While we eat, I sit with the wife. She tells me about her latest hobby – taxidermy – her passion for it absorbing, beguiling.

I talk to her, but really I watch you and V across the table. You talk, holding your wine aloft, and she watches, laughing. I can't hear what you're saying, but

I can imagine. I watch her eyes skirt your body, and I am proud, but also jealous. Not because she wants you, but because I want her to want me.

Later, we are alone in the kitchen, tidying up.
I feel her beside me, lifting the plates, slotting them carefully into the dishwasher.
We fall into a rhythm without speaking. I'm enjoying this feeling of attraction in a normal place, when she inhales.
'I have to say something,' she says.
When I look up at her, her eyes are bright.
'I've recognised you,' she says. 'From a certain website.'
'Oh really?' I fight to keep my face expressionless.
'As soon as I saw you,' she says, 'I thought, I know her. But I couldn't locate you. Then I saw him, and . . . well, the penny dropped.'
I look at her. 'So you're on it too?'
She nods.
'How long?'
'Not long,' she says.
I want to ask more, but your friend comes into the kitchen, laughing at something you've said, asking for more wine.
I find another bottle and we all return to the table.

They stay at ours, your friends in the main guest room, and her in your office, next to our room.

I settle everyone with towels. We brush our teeth, wash our faces, go to bed.

Once we're alone, I tell you.

'She recognised us from one of the websites. She's on it too.'

It takes a moment for you to realise what I mean.

'Does she look familiar?' I ask.

You shake your head. You sit up straight in bed. 'She's just next door,' you say.

I smile. 'You can't go in there.'

You grit your teeth, sigh. 'We've caught a unicorn, in our house.'

We both laugh.

'How will we see her again?'

'We'll find a way.'

She leaves a jacket behind: a purple waterproof which makes me think of walks, of her face smiling in the wind.

I message your friend to explain, to ask for her number.

A likely story, he replies, as if he knows something. He can't do.

I message her.

She's mortified of course, agrees to meet.

A container park in the city. We're late: you hurry me, not wanting her to wait alone.

The sun is trying to come out. The place is studded

with picnic benches. Around the edges, the container kitchens line up, hoping to be chosen.

I spot her before she sees us. She's frowning at her phone, weak sunlight reflecting her blonde hair. She looks up, smiles, and raises a hand.

'Sorry we're late,' I say, when we sit down. 'It was my fault.'

You smile, roll your eyes.

I straddle the picnic bench facing her, reminding myself to sit up straight.

We talk about the usual things: our jobs, the business, our lives so far. She tells us she was married, but isn't anymore. She says he cheated on her, but doesn't explain what happened. You ask, and she says it was someone at work. That she found out by reading his diary, which he left lying around, conveniently.

I try to imagine that moment of horrible revelation, of collision.

She talks openly, honestly.

When we tell her about ourselves, I feel myself trying to impress her. I talk boldly about the things we've done. *I'm different*, I'm trying to say.

I talk about want and desire and bastardise all the things I've read. *Can you want what you already have?* I make myself sound smart. She listens, and responds with her own analysis. We've read a lot of the same books, listened to the same podcasts. It's the first time I've found someone else who is as obsessed with these things as I am, and it's such a relief to talk to her.

We ask her why she's on the website, and she says she's always had a high sex drive. Her husband never wanted as much sex as her, which was why it was so hard when he had an affair.

'I want to experiment,' she says.

She tells us she's bisexual, that she had a relationship with a girl at school. I tell her about my friend, thinking it's the same thing. But hers was a real relationship, in the open, and I'm impressed by her bravery.

She asks us how long we've been doing this. A couple of years, we say. We tell her the things we've done: the first threesome, the parties, the holiday. It's easy to tell her the truth, the reality, with the good and the bad. We talk about the ghosting. I tell her about the condomless guy and it's the first time I've told anyone, even my best friend.

There is a vulnerability in this other world that is intoxicating: it is connection, more than sex, that we find here.

'I'm sorry that happened to you,' she says.

A taxi picks us up and carries us back. We're chatty in the car, but there's tension, like an elastic band stretched taut.

When we get back to her house, we meet her cat, a grumpy, pampered pet. We drink wine in the living room and I sneak peeks at the photos on the wall – family, friends – hoping to piece her together. I try to imagine this house when she lived here with her husband. I wonder if it looked different, then. I wonder if she wanted children.

Then it's happening. I'm wearing tights, a mini skirt, and we laugh as we roll them off. Under her clothes, she's strong, beautiful. When I tell her, she says she climbs. I imagine her scaling a rock face. She's really into women, into me, and her eagerness makes me unashamed of mine. We kiss on the bed while you undress, and there's something tender, but also something real. I imagine it's what it would have been like to really kiss my best friend all those years ago: a meeting of the minds, as well as bodies.

We each take turns to suck your dick, saying the right things about the size to each other, and I can feel it arouses you. There's also a sense between her and me of reading from a script, of bad dialogue in a porn film, as if we're raising one eyebrow at each other, mocking ourselves and the situation. Everything we say is true, but there's some cliché of male praise there that we're both aware of.

She touches herself as you and I kiss. It's good to have a witness, a verifier of our physicality, our attraction. I see how good she is at finding her pleasure, at getting to that place that sometimes I struggle to find. I watch her face, the noises she makes as she touches herself, and I want to be near it, to be part of it.

Afterwards, we lie together, naked. We stroke skin and talk for a long time. It feels as if we've known her for years. After a while, we leave for her guest room, and sleep.

Over the next few months, we see each other when we can.

We go to the cinema, eat popcorn, and later fuck.

We go to a scare attraction for Halloween: holding hands, taking photographs, arms around each other, other patrons streaming by. A clown runs past wielding a noisy chainsaw, chasing a screaming woman. We queue for rides, chatting, waiting for things to jump out at us. There's safety in numbers.

Sometimes, I scan the crowds around us, wondering if we'll be seen by someone we know. How would we explain?

We spend New Year together as a three. We both have other offers but choose each other. When friends and family ask us what we're doing, we say we're spending it alone, just the two of us. I want to shout from the rooftops, to tell the truth.

We drink champagne and take a bath outside. It's huge, and fits all three of us in. She and I take it in turns to be in the middle. We laugh and chat under the stars and when I look at her, I feel the buzz of something more than sex. I can see that you do too.

We go out for dinner, trying new places.

'So, what have you been up to?' she'll ask, and we'll tell her our latest stories.

'Can you keep your voices down?' she says, looking around at the other diners, mock embarrassed.

She is an audience to our secret life, a safe place we can talk about things we can't tell anyone else.

She tells us of her dating life. She's seeing a man, exploring submissiveness. She's seeing women too. She's looking for freedom, but also a safe place to come home to.

We talk about our lives: she complains about being overworked in the office, working in the evenings to get everything done. We tell her to demand more money, to say no to things. She tells me that sometimes, when she's at work, she wonders what I would do, admiring my verve, my boldness. I am startled, pleased, to be seen as the fearless person I have always wanted to be.

In the bedroom, she is the brave one. She closes her eyes, rocks her hips, as if she is steering a ship, finding her own way. We follow her. Her hair, tumbling down her back, her face flushed, the way she shudders when she finally comes. I want to be as connected to my body as she is to hers, and tell her this. We inspire each other in different ways, and I am grateful to know her.

We realise what we have is temporary, that she will find someone. We make the most of our time together, and how unique it is, to have found one person we both find attractive, whom we both trust and care for deeply. Our feelings for each other seem to compound, grow bigger, and we learn that love is not finite, but multiplies.

We go to a party together: her first.

We take photos in the apartment we've rented, you behind the camera.

We're in underwear. I take her hand, and we copy each other, listening to your prompts. *Arch your back. Turn your face. Look down.*

We drink wine and put music on. We both wear red dresses: mine makes me feel like Marilyn Monroe. Fishtail, tight-fitting, off the shoulder. Hers is shorter, fits her like a glove. You wear black tie, and we take wholesome family photos.

Inside, it's packed. I see the place through V's eyes, anew.

When it's time, I take her hand and lead her to the toilets.

Inside the stall, we change, helping each other. She's nervous: no one else is in underwear yet. I tell her we want to be first, to trust me.

When we step out into the party together, I feel the eyes follow us and I am sixteen again, with her, feeling the power of being bold.

'I see what you mean,' she whispers as we walk towards you, and I smile.

Lost Time

2022

Our friends are adrift in the sea of young children. The early fug of nappies, sleepless nights and endless screaming. The balancing of childcare and full-time jobs that are no less demanding post-procreation. The teamwork of nursery drop-offs, running noses, high temperatures, Calpol, online meetings half-attended. The days bleed into each other, a long cascade of open mouths and food and supermarkets and sorting houses. Overarched by the constant pressure to be moving up: jobs, bigger houses, extensions, gardening, cleaning, washing, ironing. Lives that were already full are now bursting open with the onslaught of new life.

The business brings a constant stream of demands too. The minutiae of the day-to-day that absorbed us at the beginning – taking bookings, marketing, cleaning, updating the website, buying stock, replenishing hand wash, toilet rolls – is now largely not our responsibility. Since opening the wedding barn, we have a larger team. We have more help, for admin and menial tasks. But with that comes the burden of leadership, of team dynamics, of human resources.

Over time, we become used to things going wrong. The more 'catastrophes' occur, the better we navigate them. The pandemic is the most obvious example: a blindside dropped out of nowhere which made us think differently, made us change things. But there are myriad small disasters every day. Once you see enough of them, you learn you can handle them. That we can handle anything.

I watch younger staff members, customers, flap and panic at the smallest things. I think: I remember that. They look to me, and I know what to say. I learn to get them to think of the solution, rather than handing it over easily. I want to give them the same thing I have learnt: that I can overcome anything.

We find a manager for the whole site who is experienced, adult, calm. Like us, he has made mistakes and understands that they are both good and bad. When I see him around the place, see the team look to him and not us, I feel a deep sense of rightness and relief. This is no longer our burden alone. He has given us the ultimate gift – a clear mind, and the energy to use it.

There is a hidden story here. One I don't tell when I'm asked how we run our business, when I'm interviewed for trade magazines or local papers. An undercurrent that is just as relevant and important, but cannot be spoken aloud.

Walking into a room of people and striking up a conversation.

Walking through a room full of people in my underwear.

Sitting at the head of a meeting table and directing a team.

Standing at the bar wearing only your shirt and talking to a stranger about politics, about anything.

Being comfortable in my views. Voicing them. Listening. Asking questions.

Pushing the boundaries in the business, trying things and getting them wrong, has increased my confidence in myself, and in us.

Pushing the boundaries in our sex lives has done the same thing, at the same time.

The snowballing of inner confidence has happened because of both: it is impossible to distinguish between them.

They are both about resilience, about being tested, about communication.

About being seen and others saying: *You are accepted. I will follow you.*

We have done these things, together. We have tested ourselves in our public lives and in our secret lives. We have found that humans are adaptable and that this is our greatest strength.

Like everything, this is about us, but it is also about you and about me.

We travel together, but also completely alone.

We witness each other's failures and successes.

We are each other's biggest supporters, always there for advice and help.

We are also each other's biggest critics. We hold each other to account.

I want you to have everything in this life. I want you to experience everything, to squeeze what we have been given hard, and not waste a single glistening drop.

You want the same for me.

We are not foolish enough to think we can offer each other everything.

Each of us must take responsibility for our wants, desires, dreams.

Again and again, we support each other.

Again and again, we choose each other.

For us, this is love.

Party

2022

We send out the invitations early in the year. Bright yellow envelopes. Inside, a colourful piece of card, designed on the business software. Feathers and a mask.

Celebrate lost time with us. Bring your A Game.
Adults only.

I imagine the invitations landing on door mats all over the country. Next to rows of kids' shoes, wellies, high heels, trainers. I imagine the slap of the letter box, our friends leaning down to pick them up.
We see them on fridges when we go to visit. People are looking forward to letting their hair down. To remembering how fun they used to be.

It is nearing the end of summer. The barn still rings with the invisible mist of communal excitement, of joy, lingering in the air. There is the smell of old places, newly renovated: old wood, sanded, varnished, made new. I love the echo my shoes make on the floor when it's empty, quiet and calm.

We spend the day getting ready: hanging bunting, stocking the bar. We have sent the team home early, wanting to prepare the place alone. We are doing the catering ourselves too: a lamb spit you are tending to outside, a huge metal frame you have built yourself, welding late into the night. The lamb will cook, turning, for hours. You baste it tenderly, patiently.

Our friends start to arrive throughout the afternoon. Some haven't been to the site yet, and I show them around. We've booked out the cottages, and soon they are full of people and noise.

It feels strange and glorious to have the run of the place at last.

You and I get ready in the house. It is a warm evening and the windows are open. I feel the last of the summer settling outside; hear our friends laughing, the chink of glasses.

I wear a feathered skirt and a beaded top. Feathers in my hair. You wear feathers stitched to short shorts, a feathered headdress. We adorn ourselves with glitter in the mirror, side by side.

We congregate at the bar, making Aperol spritzes, pouring pints from the keg.

These are friends we've collected across the years: school, university, travels, home. Some of them know what we do, and some don't. Some do what we do, and some don't. We've met some great friends on the scene: sex is like a binding agent, a catalyst to connection.

Everyone has gone all out. The ones who know but don't partake have agonised over what to wear, both wanting and not wanting to be chosen. There is a nervous electricity to the air, as everyone wonders where we will descend. I look around at all these bejewelled people and I feel power thrum. We made this happen, this party, this night, as we have so many other things.

Tell us who, my friends ask, behind their hands.

Which of us are marked out, walking amongst them?

I only smile, and shake my head. Our secret is important, but I am not ashamed. If anything, I'm proud. I want to share this world we've found, one layer beneath the surface. But I also love the mystery of being different, of keeping something to ourselves. It feels delicate, essential.

We dance, all together under glowing lights, a colourful cascade that highlights and hides. I move my body easily, freely.

She comes to find me outside.

As we used to, we share a cigarette. Remember when, we say to each other, and smile.

She asks me how my writing is going, and I tell her I've started something about our new life.

'I've written about you,' I say.

She nods, once.

'About when we were younger. Those amazing teenage years.'

She sucks on her cigarette and I am back there, at the school disco, longing for her to notice me.

How did you feel, then? I want to ask. *Did you feel the same as me?*

'Can I read it?' she says, and I nod.

Church

2022

My father's voice echoes around the stone walls, surrounding me. I look up at the wooden rafters. He sings with enthusiasm, with gusto. His voice is tuneless, beautiful.

My brother's wife walks down the aisle. She smiles wide, her pregnant stomach accentuated by her silken cream dress. I look at my brother: his smile is so pure, his eyes bright. I squeeze your hand and you smile back at me.

They've asked me to write something, to perform. When it's my turn, I walk to the front of the church, wearing jewel blue, feeling their eyes follow me. I straighten my back under their gaze, hold myself, and find my words, hearing my voice echo through the space.

> *Now, you walk together*
> *Your footsteps separate*
> *But entwining on the path*
> *When one cannot see the way ahead*
> *The other points it out*

My voice breaks: when I sit down, I look at you, and there are tears in your eyes.

The reception is at the edge of a lake, looking over the water. It's mid-winter and we wear coats, and warm ourselves inside a wide barn. Out of the long windows, we can see my brother and his bride, posing for photographs on a wooden dock.

I sip my prosecco, imagining those photos hanging in their house for years to come.

There's one of us in our spare room. We look into each other's eyes, standing in a corn field, alone. My hair is windswept and we smile at each other, as if we are the only ones there. But the photographer watched us, capturing the moment.

'You look amazing,' my mother says, squeezing my arm. 'You both do.'

I smile. 'Thanks, Mum.'

'Whatever you two are on, I want some,' she says.

If only she knew, I think.

We're called for family photos, posing in a line. We laugh at something and the photographer captures us, teeth flashing, wind tousling our hair. My sister in a sparkly dress, the bride with flowers in her hair. I hold fast onto the moment.

Later my father and I walk along the lakeside. Escaping the small talk together.

I watch myself from above, as if a bird on high.

I hear myself talk about the business, about ordinary things.

I think of him holding me aloft as a baby, examining me.

I imagine him seeing me walking through a party in my underwear.

I imagine telling him everything.

Dad, I –

I need to tell you something.

I need to explain.

We've been –

This thing is happening and I don't understand it.

It's everything you told me not to want, but I've found myself there.

I know I will never tell him.

Inside, warm with wine and happiness, I sit and listen to the speeches. I hear my brother's voice, full of hope. I see my sister bounce her baby on her knee. My parents holding hands as my brother thanks them for everything.

One day, I could destroy this with my words.

Would things ever be the same again?

Fame

2023

I send the collection of words I have collated to my writing friends.

I go to London to see them, the first time in ages.

On the train on the way there, I look out of the window.

It doesn't matter, I think. What they think doesn't matter.

'This is the best thing you've ever done,' they say.

I nod, looking for the feeling of validation, but it isn't there. For the first time, I don't need to hear their words: I have my own.

When it's almost ready, I send my book to an agent – one recommended by a friend who writes. I immediately regret it. It isn't finished, and I feel I should have waited. I should have looked at it from all angles, smoothed its rough edges. Perhaps I have ruined its chances. Perhaps I shouldn't have sent it at all.

I go into town to distract myself. I walk along the canal, watching the green water, the glass of apartments reflecting the grey sky. I'm unable to think about anything other than my book, which has left my side after all this time and is out there in the world.

I have felt this unravelling before, this handing over of something that is solely mine. I remember, lying in the park on the other side of the world, waiting and never hearing what I wanted to hear. I wonder if it will happen again. This feels different, I tell myself. But there is only one way to know.

I sit and sip coffee, eat an exquisite custard tart, trying to remind myself of pleasure, of joy. I buy myself a ring in the shape of a Venus shell, a physical reminder that whatever happens, I am enough. That the things that happened, that I have written about, are real no matter what anyone thinks about them.

I miss a call from an unknown number. Thinking it might be to do with the business, I call back.

'Hello?' The voice on the line is familiar, but I can't place it.

'Hi,' I say.

'I've just finished your book,' she says. The agent. 'I couldn't stop reading.'

The idea of the book becomes a reality. It could go out there, into the world. What would this mean for us, for our secret life?

I feel the call of the spotlight, but I don't know if I should answer. I've found this quiet, inner place. I've found autonomy, and everything I've always wanted. I shouldn't need that validated by publication.

But I want it. I am proud of what I've achieved. I want others to read it, for the things that have changed me to change them.

We talk about it. We've talked about it before, but this time, it feels real.

We discuss my parents, your parents, our staff members. I imagine walking through our business while people talk behind their hands.

This is not just my decision.

'You need to read it,' I say. It seems strange that you haven't.

'I do.' You squeeze my hand. 'But whatever you want to do, I'm with you.'

I look at you, and see your clear eyes looking back. This is a gift you're handing me. I don't know what to say.

My father and I take our annual pilgrimage to Stratford, to the theatre. He leads me proudly to the front, to the best seats, where we can see the actors' powdered faces, see them spit. We read the programme to each other.

I know, already, I will come here when he is gone and I will remember him.

In the darkness, once the play begins, we lose time together. We lose ourselves in the stories we see. In the interval, he buys ice cream, an often-repeated surprise, holding it out to me as if it is the first time.

During the second act, I glance at him – the curve of his forehead, so similar to mine. I think about his brain, how he's taught me to value mine above looks, above everything else.

Sitting side by side, I make the most of this time with him, fearful I might destroy it.

Over dinner in our favourite restaurant, he orders wine, lets me taste it.

'How's your book going?' he asks, as he always does.

'It's going well,' I say. I know this is dangerous territory. I pause. 'To be honest, Dad, I'm not sure I want to publish it.'

His eyebrows rise. 'What do you mean?'

'I mean, this book might be something I wrote for me.'

He sips his wine. 'So, you'd never show anyone?'

'I've shown my writing group.'

He nods. He knows this. 'And what did they think?'

'They think it's good.'

'So why wouldn't you want to publish it?'

How do I explain? 'It's personal, the book. I'm not sure I want people reading it.'

He nods. 'So you would finish it, and then –' He stops, unsure how to continue.

I shrug. 'Just have it for me, I suppose.'

He looks confused.

'It might affect my relationships,' I say. With you, I don't say. It might destroy all this.

I watch his face: I imagine his brain whirring over what it could be about. 'If it's about your childhood –'

'It's not,' I say. I take a sip of wine. I know I should say nothing else. 'If I published a book and asked you not to read it, would you be able to?'

He glances at me. 'I'd find it hard,' he says. 'Because I'd be proud of you. But if it was really what you wanted, I would try.'

I nod, swallow. There is a silence, and a small, mad part of me thinks of telling him everything. If I explain, perhaps . . . But I hold my nerve.

Surface

2023

We sneak away to the sun.

We get drunk on gin and tonics on the plane, raise our glasses to hard-won freedom, carved out.

We meet your friend and his new wife at the airport. He has ripped up the fabric of an ordinary life for love. We have that in common.

They work hard – frequenting the co-working space in the hotel while we run along the beach, taking our time over coffee and pastries.

When the weekend comes and they can escape their work, they are diligent about using every free moment. They book us a surf lesson, a dune buggy ride, a cooking lesson.

I am grateful, mistaking this diligence for care when it is really control.

It has nothing to do with us. They must wrestle each moment down and squeeze the juice out of it. We are observers, spectators to their efficiency.

The surf teacher is late. We wait outside the surf shop, but he doesn't materialise. She calls him – no answer.

I find a bookshop and escape the tension, delighted to find rows of left-behind holiday books, a grey-haired Englishman behind the counter.

When the teacher arrives, he is a cliché: sun-drenched, sea-battered hair, tanned skin, bright eyes. He tells us it is not his morning. He missed our booking: he is sorry. He curses his luck in Italian.

We climb into his car. There is a marathon in the town and many roads are closed. At every turn, we meet a road block. The surf teacher waves his hands out of the window.

This is not my morning, he says again.

We will go around, he says. We will find a way.

We follow a convoy of other vehicles, trying to find a way to the beach. We arrive, pull on still-damp wetsuits. We are given bright-coloured t-shirts to wear over them so we are marked out for him in the water, distinctive amongst the other surf school newbies.

On the beach, the teacher becomes serious. He describes two types of currents: what they will do to us, how to avoid them, what to do if we are under their control. I imagine drifting out to sea, a dot moving further and further away, tiring slowly. I think of sinking beneath the waves.

We lie face down on the boards in a line and he shows us how to stand as if we are in the water. I overthink each step. My body is slow-moving, heavy. The others seem to find it easy.

I feel a deep weariness descend.

I try to tell the others I will wait on the shore. They make jokes, trying to convince me.

I stay silent, but obey. I don't want to be different, but I also want to be alone.

In the water, we are at the whim of the waves. We wait for them, trying to move with them, to ride on top of them. I get used to the taste of salty water. He holds my board, directs it, tells me to paddle, when to stand. I follow instruction but without conviction. I go through the motions until we can leave the water and be on the shore again.

In the afternoon, we drive buggies across the island. You drive, I sit.

Again, I am waiting for this to end, to be alone again. I should be enjoying it, but I am not. I feel trapped by the fact that we have paid to do this, that we have to be here. I feel tired, and I long to lie in the sun with my own mind.

We have an hour to shower before dinner. I scream under the flow of water, trying to express the pent-up feeling inside. You laugh at me; we talk about it. You understand. Freedom is important to us both. We have none here, even though we are in paradise.

I ask you to fuck me. I want to be pummelled out of my frustration.

You do as I ask. We dig nails, you push me into the

bed. I want this in a specific way, and I tell you what to do. I want you to take control, but only exactly as I want you to. I want a very precise oblivion. I want you to read my mind.

I feel better, after. I feel ready for the evening ahead.

We get drunk in a tapas bar. They tell us about the first time they kissed, when he was still married.

Forbidden love is not as arousing as you think it will be, he says.

They didn't want to want each other, but they did.

There were consequences that they didn't invite in.

We talk about the day. I explain my discomfort, trying to articulate my frustration in a non-combative way.

We thought you might be feeling overwhelmed, he says.

I feel exposed, but also relieved.

Are you not exhausted? I ask him. You work so hard all week, and then you pack so much into your days off.

He looks at me and I worry I have offended him.

When I'm surfing or whatever, I can't think about anything else. I can only focus on the task at hand. I can escape my responsibilities.

I nod, understanding.

I am glad we can talk like this.

I tell them about my book. I suffer the pride in my voice for the sake of impressing them.

We have the same conversation I've had before, many times.

Whether I should publish it. What the repercussions of that would be.

I want their views to unlock something within me, to solve the problem.

Their words feel hollow, without substance.

I have asked for their opinion but feel trapped by it.

When they talk about it, I feel myself close like a clam.

I realise that no one can give me the answer.

Angel

2023

There is a golden angel, sitting on top of a column in the middle of the square.

I only notice her once I'm seated in the sun. I can see the river, beyond the wide stone wall, the boats that move past, ferrying tourists who point cameras at Notre Dame. The waiter comes and I order coffee. He nods, and turns away.

I slip a cigarette out of my bag, long and thin and so Parisian, and light it, smiling as I breathe in.

I am in Paris to finish the book. I am completely alone with my own mind, at last.

Before I came here, I suggested that you meet V alone. At first, you were surprised. I explained my reasons. It is a new frontier, one we have been evolving towards. I am beginning to feel I would like to stand alone, to test myself without you beside me. Perhaps it would be easier to pursue my own desires without considering yours. I want to see how I would feel if you did the same. Paris is a good time to try it: I will be absorbed in the book, distracted by the task at hand, by my favourite city. You will be lonely without me.

'I promise that if I feel strange, or regretful, I'll let you know,' I say.

We discuss communication, how much I want to know. I can't be sure of the answers, but I promise to speak up. I ask you not to tell me anything unless I request it.

When you realise I'm serious, you propose it in the group chat. I also message her privately, to let her know that I'm fine with it, and that if I'm not, I'll let them know. She tells me she has so much respect for our relationship that she'll take the lead from us. I say we will also consider her: that her feelings are just as important.

You arrange to meet.

I wake and I write. The book takes shape easily, almost without effort, as if it is meant to come to life.

When I grow tired, I walk the streets of Paris. I follow the river. Every time I see the Eiffel Tower, my heart rises and I smile. I drink coffee and feel the sun on my face. I follow the flow of the city, the green man lighting my way as I cross the road. I drink wine and eat dinner alone. I wander through art galleries, feeling my mind still in the presence of someone else's creation. I do exactly as I please.

Now that the work has been seen, I see it differently.

I am leaping inside with the joy of praise. My words have weight, have form, mean something.

When I write now, I am sure of myself. That tremulous thread of doubt is gone. It feels so good.

I float around Paris, living inside it. My mind jumps ahead, to the world reading my words, to what I might receive in return. I imagine myself on-stage, on panels, smiling under the lights while people look at me. It is hard not to get carried away with the wave of a future that doesn't exist.

I become anxious about anonymity and try to hide us within the story. I create a bakery we buy instead of holiday cottages, and add metaphors of kneading dough, to symbolise struggle, making things out of nothing, creativity, and the human body. I metaphorise everything. I bastardise reality.

I think of the reader, and I write for them and not for me.

I think of whoever is reading this, and I worry about their judgement, and I need to make them understand what happened within my marriage. I try to answer questions which perhaps there are no answers to.

All the training I have had rises up to meet me. I need to show, not tell. I can't be speaking to you directly like this. I can't say clearly what I really mean.

I smooth every sentence. I rewrite, removing the essence of the real. I remove any rough edges that may cause splinters, and in doing so, I remove what is great about what I have done.

*

When I read it back, nothing rings true. I know it's not how it's supposed to be.

The writing felt too easy because it was too easy.

I go back into the work. I strip it back. I try to be more vulnerable, to tell the truth.

I take a deep breath and try to return to the quiet part of myself. The questioning part.

I try to remember where the book came from, before there was a reader.

I forget about the rules.

On the night when you meet V, I take myself out for dinner, sitting in a French bistro. I hear the sounds of foreign voices, and I eat delicious food. I drink a glass of red wine.

I feel a quiet contentment. I wonder what you're doing, at this moment, but I don't feel anything other than curiosity. I wait for other feelings to arise, but they don't. I go home and eat a bar of chocolate, write a few more lines. In bed that night, I make myself come.

The next day, I call you. You tell me it went well.

'Are you going to run away with her?' I say, lightly.

You laugh. 'Now why would I do that?'

On my last day, I go to the Sacré-Cœur. It is my favourite place, the city laid out like a mirage below.

I tell myself that what happens with the book doesn't matter. The book is my best attempt to chart something deeply personal. The book is a by-product, not the experience itself.

I remember coming here before I found you. I sat in the deserted carousel at the foot of the steps and cried as I finished *Vanity Fair*. I longed for a life of adventure, of words. I longed for a love like we have. One that has no edges, no boundaries. I couldn't have imagined how it would feel, to be held up, but also to be free to fly.

Chaos

2023

This city – chaos under a beating sun. Graffitied metal shop shutters, splashes of colour that stay inside the lines. We roll down the windows of the taxi, feeling the warm air rush past our skin.

Cafés spill out onto the street, music plays.

Along the promenade, people glide by on scooters and rollerblades as if they were teenagers. We walk in the last of the sun, the heat still pressing, softly, all around us. Expose yourself, the sunlight seems to say, let me look at you, let me touch you.

We feel the eyes of others graze our bodies, meet our eyes. Here, we blend, we fit. It feels so good.

Follow the rules, the tannoy voice says.

People strip off their clothes, lie naked on the sand. We do too, laying out a colourful sheet to flatten ourselves on. There is nothing to do but look at the sky, walk to the water. Eyes land on us as we stand, step towards the sea.

I love to float, far out, unseen, and watch the beach

from far away. The people, sitting, standing, walking, watching. I am here, amongst them, one of them.

You like to stand at the water's edge, your body on display. I think of peacocks, of marble-sculpted men, circled in the museum. The eyes on you are fire and you burn at being seen.

At night, the sun still on our skin, we shower to remove the sand, the cloy of the day. We dress in colourful clothes we couldn't wear at home. We take photos of each other, staring out of the balcony at the busy rush of streets below. Staring down the camera. We take them for ourselves, but also for the others who will see them online. A marketing campaign we curate together.

Braless, I walk the streets, your hand in mine. I feel the eyes, and raise myself to meet them. We find one of many bars and sit street-side: watching people pass, and discussing who we like. We search, on apps, and find others trying to catch the moment, to live inside it.

Padrón peppers, slivers of silver-white anchovies, bread slathered with tomato, garlic. We eat less: the flavours pop inside our mouths. We drink wine and cheers to us, to our place, found.

The club is invisible to the street. We follow directions on your phone, down residential streets that suggest nothing. I think of early dates: your hand-drawn maps, how you planned all that for me. I follow you again, floating off course in the most delicious way. You ring the bell: a door opens. Inside, a small porch, another door with an eye-height letter box which slides open. Male kohl-lined eyes blink, speak Spanish.

'We're looking for the club,' you say.

One blink more, and the door opens. A counter, a screen, a cloakroom for coats. We pay admission, are ushered inside.

'Do you want to change, or wait awhile?'

We stay in ordinary clothes, for now. Beyond the door, there is a long crowded bar. The people wear stockings, latex, fishnets, chains: men, women, somewhere in between. Nothing matters here, and there is freedom rising in the air like smoke.

I'm overdressed in a tiny mini skirt and top, but feel at home at once. You wear jeans, a t-shirt: we stand out, but order drinks and wait.

They find you where we sit and draw you in, taking your hand. I watch them take off your clothes, delicately. They marvel at your body underneath, their hands moving slowly as if enjoying you. I sit beside and watch, and you look at me, eyes wide. I nod, and see you harden, at me seeing all of you, with them.

I feel so proud and full of love for everyone in this room. For seeing you in ways I can't, as new. I see you differently, as mine.

Another night, we meet for cocktails at a roadside bar. Neon lights, fairground-like, flare across the interpass.

A promenade of trees arches over us, as we study an intricate menu.

I choose something tart and fresh, wanting to feel clean, and we wait for them to arrive.

As soon as I see them, I know it will be one of those evenings where I take, not give. He is short and very American: clean cut, as if under his clothes, I will find smooth plastic between his legs. She is poised and beautiful, but in a hands-off way, like an ornament, waiting on a shelf.

I am not immediately attracted to them, but I no longer expect this, understanding how rare an immediate lightning bolt is. I also know to wait and see, that sometimes want can grow into real connection. If it doesn't appear, I know I can find my own pleasure, not expecting to be dragged along by attraction, by want, by the other person. I will take control of my own evening.

We talk about our vanilla lives, connected already by secrets we hold.

He is a Navy man, and talks of ships, of working away. I imagine him in uniform and still feel nothing.

She is a writer too, but not the interesting kind. She writes for money, to avoid failing at the real thing.

We tell stories of our lives: living overseas, the cottages, the wedding barn. And now this new city.

You're brave, they say, and we look at each other and laugh.

When the drinks are done, we make a plan: flag a taxi to a place they know.

A gated house, high in the hills. Large sandy mansions, behind tall walls, shaded by plants I don't know the name of.

At the entrance, we pass over our belongings, are handed towels, and change into lingerie. He touches my exposed nipple, and already, it feels wrong.

But I show willing, taking him in my mouth. I'm good at this now, and know it, taking pleasure from the noises he makes. *Fuck*, he says, and I speed up, swallowing him deeper, slowly showing him what I can do.

He is grateful, and wants to return the favour. I close my eyes, breathing deep, and fill my body with only this moment. I let the sensation take over, and without thinking, float away. It is easy now, and different, to find this place I know so well. I move my own body, rubbing myself against his face, not thinking of him at all.

'Fuck that was hot,' he says, kissing me, and I smile at the irony of it. Finding myself is the hottest thing of all.

You and I wake late, the sounds of this new city rumbling through our sleep.

The warmth of the day is just beginning, light glowing through the green leaves of a banana plant on the balcony. Beyond that, the sunlit warmth of old walls.

We dress, walking through shady streets. We find a secret garden and share late breakfast.

In the afternoon we sleep again, under a twisting fan, hearing voices echo from the street below.

I look across at you, the white sheet draped across your taut brown body.

Our roots are deep and we grow, green and bright, into the sunshine of a new day.

Her

2023

I send her my book. Almost immediately, I regret it.

What if I misread things, all those years ago? What if I jeopardise our friendship, now?

I worry that she will not like the version of herself I have put on paper.

The form of my worry is large and hollow. It follows two steps behind me. I am aware of it, but it is also nothing.

She tries to call me but I miss her.

I try to call back. Twice.

She has the power, though I am the person with the narrative.

I have opened the door to the place I am in control of, the place that is mine alone.

When we speak, she says everything I want her to.

She underlines things she likes and sends me screenshots of them.

I ask her if she remembers things how I do, and she says she does.

I should feel validation, but I surprise myself by not feeling anything.

Her words feel like they have nothing to do with me.

They are inconsequential when I thought they would be everything.

They are disappointing.

It makes me wonder what I want from this. From people reading it.

Windows

2023

They usher me into a glass room.

They pour coffee, pass a small milk jug.

I dot milk on the table and long to rub at it with my fingers.

I have longed to sit in a room like this, high up above the city, surrounded by books. I have longed for important people to read my work. To hold it up to the light and cast it worthy. To say they want to publish it.

It feels so exactly like my imaginings that I wonder if this is a dream.

I smile to myself, thinking how clichéd it would be if it was. *She woke up and it was all a dream.*

They begin. The praise should nourish. It should be everything. I have waited for it for so long.

I had predicted I would feel relief, that the dark hole inside me would seal and close. I had predicted feeling thrilled. Instead, I feel serene. I feel calm as I watch their mouths move. I feel a cool and calming nothing.

I am both powerful and completely helpless at the exact same time.

*

It is the strangest thing to hear them talk about things we have done, in this clean ordinary space. It is surreal that I have sent these private things out into the world.

I am still not certain it was the right thing to do.

The joy comes later. When I am going about my day, picking up a coffee on the way to meet you across town. Riding the Tube amongst the throng of everyday.

The words they said in that glass room come back and I smile that they were really spoken aloud.

I will hold my book in my hands.

I am proud of this thing I have created.

It will go out into the world, and I will watch it float away.

Early afternoon, you and I walk through the city to Borough Market. There is the sizzle of pans, the smell of hot cheese, of chestnuts.

We stop at the oyster stall. You queue, ordering wine and oysters, chatting to the man about which ones he recommends. You are probably telling him about the business. I see him throw back his head, laugh, and watch you smile.

You bring back your spoils and we rest them on a barrel. The wine is sharp and wakes me up. We cheers, tipping oysters into our throats. The saltiness, the slipperiness. I want more and more.

Christmas is coming and the city is readying itself.

The lights twinkle, the shop windows glow with gold and red. I take your hand as we walk through it together, through streets crowded with other people. Your hand is warm in mine.

Back in the hotel room, I take a long hot shower. Naked, I stand in front of floor-length glass windows looking out over the city, as day turns to night.

I watch the sky turn deeper blue, the lights come out, each one a sign of life.

I watch the cars drive, stop, move on.

People waiting inside, going somewhere.

You sleep in the plush hotel bed behind me, steeling yourself for the night ahead.

There is the fizz of anticipation. Of walking into a room of people we don't know. Of talking to them. Of looking around, making a selection. Drawing them towards us, a careful, expert dance. We will take our clothes off, and I will feel eyes on me again. I will do exactly what I want.

I am beginning to know now what this is. What I am attracted to, and what I'm not. I learn to feel my way through each new situation.

We meet people; I either like them or I don't. I don't try to convince myself of anything.

I am the subject. I am active in our real life. I lead. I am not ashamed of being proud of our business, of what we have achieved.

And in our secret lives, too, I practise this. I say *I'm not feeling this* out loud.

I am not always strong. I take each moment as it comes.

I have found a fire within myself, and I want to fan it, to see it light me up inside.

We meet them in a bar before the party. Four couples.

There's a theme – boho chic. I'm wearing a crochet dress I bought in Portugal, with gold underwear.

I notice him across the group. He's tall with dark hair. Broad shoulders, wide lips. When he smiles, his teeth are white and straight. He reminds me of the men my best friend dated at university, who played high-level university sport, at home on a playing field, in the showers.

We are playing our parts, telling them the story of us.

I watch you talk, telling them about Australia, your job in the outback. I talk about being a writer, and they ask what my books are about, if they would have heard of them.

We are good at this, at setting out our stall together. We make a display of who we are, of how much we love each other, to attract others. *We are different*, we say. *Join us.*

I smile at him; he is surprised, smiles back.

At the party, we know people. The DJ, some couples we've played with before. A single girl we had fun with at an orgy. We greet them like old friends, kissing on both cheeks.

I dance in my underwear. I feel his eyes on me and know something will happen.

I go to the toilet, up some stairs, out of sight.

I feel him follow me.

I'm talking to someone in the corridor when I feel his hand in mine, pulling me away.

He pushes me up against the wall and kisses me.

It is a good kiss, full of the waiting between us. I want to get under his shirt. His hands are all over me.

This is it, I think.

I want more of this. I want to see him again. Alone. This is the first time I've thought this.

I will talk to you about it, I think.

I feel the creak of a new door opening.

Another finish line we'll pass, into an unknown place, where we'll stand together and alone.

Epilogue

Everything and Nothing

The town is waking, blinking in the early light. Awnings are still shut, there are no other footsteps in the cobbled streets. I run past the shuttered church, towards the bay, my feet on stone. Boats rock softly, silently, in the harbour.

I take the rising road, the town slipping away. My lungs expand, drawing more air: into me, and out again. The light applies warm pressure and I feel my muscles stretch, moving me through this moment, towards the next.

Below me: cliffs begin to spread, rock pools glimmer with green water.

The road now slopes downward. The curve of a soft flat beach lies waiting. I step carefully over the rocks and clamber down, filled with the calm thrill of being alone, as if this place belongs to me.

I strip off my clothes at the water's edge. For a moment, I look up at the path I've travelled to see if you have followed me. I look briefly along the shoreline, for early-morning eyes, but there is no one there.

I step into the water, levelling my breath against the cold. I stop when the water is mid-thigh. I see: the false solidity of water stretching out, curved sunlight, the silver of a passing fish. I breathe in, put my hand on my chest. Then step forwards, and I am under, the water muffling my ears, covering me. I float on my back. I blink at the sun. I think of doing this as a child, both in and out of the world, my parents somewhere on the beach. I think of all the moments that have passed, and this one too, and how too soon, they will be gone. How all I really have is this one, now. I float, weightless, everything and nothing, all at once.

Acknowledgments

As I write in these pages, this book is more than a book to me: it is a by-product of my experiences and will therefore always be immensely special. I am so grateful to have had the opportunity to capture some part of life and for others to read it and, I hope, take something from it.

I would like to thank my family and friends, both those who know and those who do not, for enriching my life. Thank you to everyone we have met on the scene for some scintillating experiences, and also for being brave and vulnerable enough to seek out your true selves. To the organisers of the various events we attend, thank you for creating a safe, extravagant, beautiful setting for us to live out our wildest and mildest fantasies.

Thank you to my writing group for always being the first sounding board, and for being more interesting than the best novel. Thank you to my agent for her enthusiasm, intelligence, and balls. Thank you to all at Michael Joseph for making this book a reality.

Thank you to V – we love you. Thank you to her, for inspiring me to live a big life. Thank you to you, for being by my side, always.